Goodbye Fatness,
Hello Gorgeous!

Goodbye Fatness, Hello Gorgeous!

Tips and Tricks for Overcoming Healthy Eating Obstacles

LORI M. SWEENEY

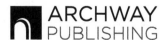

As with any diet or eating/exercise program, please consult your doctor of medical professional/healthcare provider of choice before proceeding with any advice offered in this book. The author, publishers, and distributors of this book are not responsible for negative effects or aspects that result from following book advice. They are not liable for damage or negative consequences that result from following any aspect of this book.

This book is sold with an understanding that the author, publishers, and distributors are not responsible for any detrimental effects as a result of the information presented in this book. No warranties or guarantees are for any physical, psychological, emotional, financial, or even commercial damages. Information in this book is not to be utilized as an alternative to medical advice.

Archway Publishing books may be ordered through booksellers or by contacting:

Archway Publishing
1663 Liberty Drive
Bloomington, IN 47403
www.archwaypublishing.com
1-(888)-242-5904

Because of the dynamic nature of the Internet, any web addresses or links contained in this book may have changed since publication and may no longer be valid. The views expressed in this work are solely those of the author and do not necessarily reflect the views of the publisher, and the publisher hereby disclaims any responsibility for them.

Any people depicted in stock imagery provided by Thinkstock are models, and such images are being used for illustrative purposes only. Certain stock imagery © Thinkstock.

ISBN: 978-1-4808-1246-8 (sc)
ISBN: 978-1-4808-1247-5 (e)

Library of Congress Control Number: 2014918640

Printed in the United States of America.

Archway Publishing rev. date: 11/12/2014

Acknowledgements

I would like to thank my parents Joe and Dorothy for believing in me and seeing my good qualities way before I ever could. I would like to thank them for their patience in handling a girl who had low self esteem. They always encouraged me and were more than just parents. They were my true friends who were amazing, giving people. Their hardships were worse than average and I admire them for their positive spirit and perseverance.

I am truly grateful to my husband Robert and now eleven year old son (going on 30) Joseph. Both supported me through all hardships and my weight loss journey. My son has been a source of tremendous strength, encouraging me along the way. He is so proud that he even told many he encountered about my significant weight loss. Such praise along with encouragement fueled me on this journey and I will be forever grateful.

To my dear friend Mohammed who is like a true brother to me. You are kind, giving, and charitable. You have been there for me to celebrate victories and to help me through the rough times. Good people are tough to find and I want to make sure you remain in this world. Health is important to me and I want to help you get well.

I would like to thank the writers/reporters who wrote amazing articles that truly captured my story. They all worked hard on every detail and put their hearts into their work. As a result, they were able to tell my story well and inspire others as a result. So thank you Michal Kapral, Chuck O'Donnell, Janelle Griffith, and Shapefit.com.

I would like to thank the members and staff of the YMCA; I began my weight loss journey there. The kind, motivational words they offered me were so helpful and meaningful. I also thank them for posting my articles to motivate others, which is one of my primary goals.

Contents

Home Luggage

Luggage You Need For Venturing Out

The Dining Out Chapter Series

More cool stuff

Preface

There I was standing on the set of a major television show in clothes I never thought I could wear in my lifetime. I was in a skirt (a little too mini for my taste) and a gorgeous sweater, so proud to be posing. I was in heels, something I would never wear when I was overweight because of fear that those skinny sticks would snap from my 272 pound weight. I actually had to practice walking up and down the halls of the studio in order to get used to the high heels. After much practicing, I was able to master the walk and did well. The audience cheered and I stood there beaming. While up there, front and center, I bubbled over with gratitude to have such an opportunity to be seen by millions. I could set an example for many, many people who suffer as I did. So many are overweight, which could lead to cruel words and prejudices. And this overweight body I had also limited friendships and everyday physical activities. But with my hard work and strategies, I became a thin person with a positive spirit. I changed my body and mindset, which led to amazing things I never imagined. The physical transformation led to the mental transformation. Feeling good and wanting to tutor on a wider scale, I share my tips and tricks with you.

This is not where I thought I would end up. In fact, my naysayers would never expect "Lori the Loser" to do anything great. They would never believe that I shaped up and was on a show in which the host called me "saucy," a response to my sexy posing. I was the fat slob, the reject, the joke. No one wanted to know me at all. There was torture on a daily basis. It existed in my neighborhood, in school, in day camp, in dancing school, and even in my family. Such negative words every single day, along with some physical abuse, led a life of a recluse. I had self-hate and was not outgoing at all. I looked at the ground a lot, being ashamed of myself. I was indeed the loser and was reminded of that so often. After all that, I morphed into a slimmer, confident being who is now able to hold her head up high.

While other models chattered on about being nervous to even walk on set, I was ready to face it bravely. The recluse no longer existed and was long gone. Walking on and posing as the cameras filmed us made it an incredible experience. There was no fear and I felt comfortable "onstage" as if it was my home. With such a feeling, I knew I came a long way.

When the show aired, I was called "saucy lady" by friends because of the host's comment. So I went from shy, to saucy, from obese to thin. My opportunities did not end with that show. Since then, my story has been getting out into the world slowly but steady. In the May 2014 issue of *Oxygen Magazine*, a feature article titled me "The Biggest Winner." *The Hillsborough Beacon* generously published an almost full page piece. *The Star Ledger*, one of the largest newspapers in New Jersey, put me on the front page, "above the fold" and just under the newspaper's title. That story was located on the front of the Health Section and was two pages long. Shapefit. com, a fitness website, did a story on me which included incredible detail and great positioning of "before" and "after" pictures. Though touting such facts, I am not a braggart. I am humble and proud. Someone like me made it in print and on the internet. I also made it into the hearts of many. Many of those kind hearts have phoned the newspapers, asking when my book is coming out. I have worked hard to pair problems with solutions and am proud to present these to you!

I am enjoying the fruits of my labor that I never thought possible. So I share my tips and tricks so you could say *Goodbye Fatness, Hello Gorgeous!*

Introduction

Have you ever seen slogans or sayings denouncing the dreaded diet? I remember seeing a poster which displayed "diet" is "die" with a "t" on the end. I have also seen and heard the word "diet" to be a four letter word, equivalent to a curse. When I wanted to lose weight for that reunion, wedding, party, or vacation, I dreaded what had to be done in order to get down those pounds. It was indeed perceived as a grueling task, involving eating yucky, packaged diet foods, doing mundane exercises, and depriving myself of "the good stuff" while others indulge. Losing/maintaining weight does not have to be a chore, yet most of us make it into horrid experiences. If "dieting" is unpleasant, we can only have the patience for so long and we end up quitting. If something is not "enjoyable" or semi - doable, it is difficult to stick to it. Therefore, drop the diet and pick up "healthy living!" This has to be a change that is a forever thing. Crazy diets and gross diet foods will either lead to temporary success or complete failure. You need a forever tool that can be achieved day after day with success most of the time. The plan also has to be remotely "fun." That is where my plan comes into the picture. It is more than a tool, but is a collection of "tools" to handle what temptations, bad habits, or situations we face in life that lead us to unhealthy eating. More importantly, it is "doable" and in some aspects, fun!

This lifestyle change has to be feasible, not taxing or punishing. My plan gives you the tools you need, no matter where you may be. The beauty of this book is that it can be used for every healthy eating plan. Tips and tricks will help you stick to your plan without the external factors negatively impacting your efforts. Challenges to stay on the healthy eating path occur both inside and outside the home. We have to learn to overcome these challenges or obstacles while making it semi enjoyable. We are therefore going to make life/healthy eating a vacation, not an abominable chore. I will present you with three different "suitcases." When you go on vacation, you at least bring one suitcase that holds what you need while at your destination. My suitcases will provide you with what you need for two major locations: home (your staycation), venturing out (restaurants, holiday parties, work). In each suitcase are tips and tricks to handle any "world" you travel to throughout the day. These items in each case will come in handy, some more than others, depending on destination and lifestyle. Keep in mind that sometimes items can be in more than one case. For instance, you make sure you bring the cell phone when traveling to work or traveling on vacation. Therefore, commonalities can be found in some of the luggage, and as a result, I present you with a third piece of baggage, your core suitcase. This is what you need to have with you at all times, whether inside or outside the home.

This approach worked for me. It took me three and a half years to lose 125 pounds, and I have maintained for many years. After a time, the tools will become a part of your life, as they are of mine, and will become second nature. You will get to automatically know what is needed and will choose the right tools to utilize. With a positive spirit and the drive to succeed and make healthy eating more fun than a chore, you will program yourself to have success in life.

Who am I besides the one who lost all that weight? Well, to

know me is to understand that I am an average person who has always loved helping people. I tried to be a friend to those who wanted one. I tried to educate people, whether it was as a scientist, teacher, tutor, friend, spouse, or mom. My soul is special, but my body is not; it is just like everyone else's. I was not blessed with a fast metabolism. Everything I eat has an effect on me, especially when it comes to my hips and abdomen. I do not come from a family of thin people, so "thin" is definitely not strong in my genetics. I was not thin all of my life. For most of my years, I was overweight and then became morbidly obese. After trying to lose weight, and of course failing several times over, I finally found something that works. I did not hire a personal chef to cook healthy meals, nor did I utilize a personal trainer. I did not even temporarily use a trainer to help tone me. My results solely come from me. Aside from getting two knee surgeries as a result of a careless driver, I did not get additional surgeries, especially those for weight loss. I also did not have cosmetic surgery. My successes have solely been my own and I did not utilize a magic potion, powder, or pill to reach my goals.

I was not always so independent and tried the latest products to help me in my weight loss journey over the years. I tried a lot of diet plans, pills, powders, and contraptions. Most of the promises were empty. Infomercials seemed to guarantee a way to get me to reach my weight loss goal. When the product arrived, I was sorely disappointed; these products never delivered. Another avenue I tried was the weight loss clinic, a place where I would be coached, encouraged, and educated. Some weight loss clinics that I tried promised a caring staff, yet they were practically pushing me out the door. I was not asked how my week went, or if I faced any challenges. If questions were asked, annoying countenances were displayed. I would either get a quick answer or an eye roll as I was hurried. After all, appointment times were close to each other, so the employee couldn't wait to get rid of me in order to get to the next appointment. I was quickly weighed, asked to choose the products I wanted for the week, and then hustled out the door. As one can see, there was no consultation or coaching of any kind. There was no genuine interest or concern for a client struggling to reach goals. I was on my own to fail miserably.

I was tired of products that did not work. I was tired of the cycle of trying and failing. Additionally, I was tired of fat jokes, restrictions, and naysayers telling me that I will never lose weight. My job as a scientist trained me to always try to figure out what is wrong, to derive a hypothesis. This was my approach to my recent weight loss. Why did I keep failing? What triggered me to stray from healthy eating? After identifying factors that made me weak, that made me fail, I came up with my own program. I identified problems and came up with solutions. For the first time in my life, I see success. The three and a half years to lose the desired weight and reach goal is a reasonable time. It is wise to take the weight off slowly. This slow pace prevented me from having to face loose skin. My body was able to adapt as the pounds were dropped slowly, and the surgery to remove loose skin was not at all needed. As a result of losing 125 pounds, I went from a jeans size 26 to a size 4. My shirt size was a 3X, but is now a size small. Such a dramatic loss has changed my life for the better, and I am enjoying more rewards than I even imagined. Success is endless and is enjoyed daily. Therefore, it is with great pride that I present *Goodbye Fatness, Hello Gorgeous!*

I say goodbye to diets because it is the diet that is short lived. As previously mentioned, diets are associated with stresses, hardships, and failures. People give up their favorite foods or ingredients, instructed in some way to never eat them again. Some do abnormal things like drink special shakes or eat frozen, canned, or astronaut food. These things cannot last forever and patience wanes, leading to individuals to return to their normal eating habits. After this surrender, people gain weight or stay their same overweight/

obese selves. We truly have to bid farewell to dieting. The diets are temporary; what we need on a "forever basis" are good eating habits. We have to make great choices every day, learning how to cope with challenges that come our way.

So keep in mind that this book can help you regardless of the eating plan. You can have the best, most healthy eating plan in the world, consuming all the right foods in the right amounts, and even incorporating exercise. It seems like a great plan until internal and external factors ruin efforts. Certain tips and tricks can benefit children too. Of course such must be utilized with parental and physician/health care provider discretion. The lives of children sometimes run parallel to those of adults. That is, the same external factors cause overeating. When I was a child, I did not know how to handle stress eating, holidays, restaurants, movie theater food, and food portions. There was no measuring of the foods in my home, unless it was for some kind of recipe! The percent of overweight children has increased over the years, which tells me that such tips and tricks are so needed. A lot of great approaches such as those I offer in this book, as well as good eating habits, can indeed be incorporated into young lives, making significant differences. My book helps overcome hurdles that may hamper healthy eating success. What are some of these factors? Here is a sampling:

- Friends/relatives who push food on you
- "Munchee" attacks
- Your lifestyle forces you to eat on the go.
- A string of holidays
- A string of parties
- Eating too fast
- Dining out
- Negative People who chide efforts
- Parties in general

- Lack of time/time crunches
- Tremendous stress
- Free food/samples
- Going to the movies
- Excuses
- Work in general
- Gross diet food
- Crazy diets that are too limiting

These are just a few things that can ruin an attempted healthy lifestyle. For some people, these factors hold people back, impeding progress. In other circumstances, people quit altogether. I can help you overcome such hurdles and stay on the healthy track.

The best way to get the most of this book is to take notes. Dedicate a spiral notebook and use that exclusively for your notes. We can all be so forgetful! Or, photocopy my **Notes of Success** located in the back of this book to write down all the new approaches you will use for each of your destinations. You can take notes and bring the sheets with you on your various destinations to remind you of the tips and tricks that are important to utilize. If you are like me in my "old" age, you tend to forget good ideas. I keep telling myself that I will remember, and then I forget. I honestly have a lot of tips to offer, so writing them down would be best. Keeping such an organized journal of good ideas/tips will help you tremendously. More importantly, implement these ideas/tips into your life. The book is divided into sections of how to handle challenges at home, and outside ventures, including work. Sections could be selected, depending on the "world" you are going to visit or be in the most.

The tips that made me successful did not only help me with my food intake and exercise. Most diet books go right to the food tips. I start with the mindset; that is the most important. If we do not have the right frame of mind, a healthy eating lifestyle will not last for long. Be prepared to change this mindset and have an ambitious, fresh approach. Advice about how to handle external factors follows. There are also great recipes throughout the book that are versatile. So collectively, this book will help you with your mind, spirit, food, exercise, and outside pressures that cause your foundation to crumble.

Losing weight and staying in shape takes a lot of work and overall effort. We are worth it, though! If I can work 50 to 60 hours a week, take time for family and friends, and take time to keep in shape, you can too. We have to make ourselves, our health in particular, a priority. After all, aren't we worth it? I think so! We have to take care of ourselves, not just for us, but for our family, friends, and even for the sometimes dreaded workplace! Remember, you come first. You are important and have to do what is best for your health. So be kind to yourself - like and even love yourself. If not, you will not persevere as you should, so it is important to fight for a better "you".

Follow my advice, take the time, make the effort, approach with vigor and an open mind. Doing so will allow you to say goodbye to fatness and hello to gorgeous!

CHAPTER 1

How I Got This Way

Before we go to our suitcases, it is important for you to know who I am and how I got this way. You will see that things never came easy for me. Sadly, life was far from normal; my childhood was hell, and no one seemed to believe in me or give me a chance at friendship. An entire neighborhood shunned me for many reasons, mainly for being overweight. My hair also added to my oddity. Unfortunately, no one who worked in the local hair salons knew how to cut my thick, curly hair. It was the 1970's when thin, flowing hair was "in." Therefore, every haircut was awful and I always looked odd. My hair was wild and puffy, which made me look like a person who hadn't brushed her hair in ages. My clothes were so baggy and awful looking. My mom was limited in clothing options. My pants were elastic polyester pants. Jeans were not an option because they were too fitted. I was always gaining weight and had to have clothes that had more "give." My appearance made my childhood very lonely. I was shunned and teased oftentimes to the point of tears. To make matters worse, I had no sibling interaction. My brothers were ten plus years older than me and did not have time to give to their little sister; they were always out with friends. Other relatives were not supportive either. For years, two relatives used to chant, "I don't want her, you can have her, she's too fat for me," and then laugh hysterically after their taunts made me cry.

The only comforts I had in my life were my parents, my toys, and lots of food. Eating special treats was a way to make pains go away or to at least feel better for a short period of time. Treats at home included cakes, cookies, chips, and lots of candy. Soda was the prominent beverage in the house, especially Coca Cola, Tab, and Fresca. Drinking water was unheard of in my home. Tap water was horrible tasting and fancy water filters were not highly commercialized during this time. My parents thought it was awfully expensive to pay for bottled water. Therefore, juice was the morning beverage and soda was the main drink for the rest of the day. Food was a huge comfort, and I learned to reward myself with food if I was ever blue. If my dad saw I was unhappy, a visit to the ice cream shop was in order. If I had a bad day, a trip to some fast food joint was my reward to cheer me up. From this, I learned that eating food, lots of it, was the only way to alleviate the pain I had in my life. Therefore, I would medicate myself with food.

Mom worried about me eating, but was more concerned that I did not eat enough! I had to clean my plate at every meal - not leaving a morsel of food behind! Mom made sure there were lots of snacks in the house, and many were not healthy, especially when I ate them in mass quantities! Bags of potato chips, corn chips, and other "niceties" were readily available on the kitchen counter. Candy bars were placed in that special drawer so I could dig into the stash whenever I wanted. Sometimes she would buy special pastries that she knew I liked if she ventured out somewhere special. Mom even worried about my eating through adulthood. I remember how she would call me at work after my lunch break to ask me if I ate lunch that day. She always inquired about what I had to eat. Because I ate a great deal, my answers always satisfied her and she was glad that I had enough to eat.

I know it seems like my parents were bad people, but they truly were not. Both of my parents tried to make me happy in my miserable life. They did wonderful things and tried to say words of encouragement. Of course I did not believe the latter because, after all, they were my parents. In my heart, I felt they were biased because I was their daughter, so their comments were discounted. Instead, I chose to believe the words of my nemeses, those who would say horrible things that would cripple my confidence and my spirit. I also believed people's actions and felt they were justified because after all, I was a horrible person. People shunned me for my tan skin, geeky appearance, and "fatness;" it did not matter if I was a good person or not. Just being an overweight kid was enough for people to avoid me completely, never giving me a chance for friendship. It was horrible to be either ignored or taunted. So many people put me down over the years; it ate away at my confidence until barely any was left. I chose to take in their words, to absorb their words, and to hate myself. Food seemed to be one of my primary friends. It was the only way my parents could make me happy. They gladly obliged because it was the only way for them to be successful in cheering me up.

The satisfaction from the fattening treats was short term, but the weight gain from such foods was long term. Being overweight caused particular problems throughout my elementary, junior high, and high school years. Sometimes I was hit or shoved for being a "fat loser." Children enjoyed making fun of me. People bullied me primarily because I was very heavy. What hurt me even more was that bullying was done in front of teachers, who did nothing to stop it. Sometimes it was the main event in the classroom. A bunch of students would taunt me, yelling insults at me and teachers would say nothing. Those who did not join in simply watched and enjoyed the show. Teachers would stand and look at the scenario, never intervening. Some would not even interrupt the verbal attacks in order to begin class! They patiently waited until students were finished insulting me.

One year I had a study hall that I initially looked forward to so I could finish studying and school work. It was difficult to concentrate when two bullies insulted me. I was always called fat and ugly. I was compared to an elephant, a hippopotamus, a yak, and a pig. The study hall teacher allowed this to go on. It was another show for people to see without interruption. My dad died in his sleep that year, a result of a massive heart attack. I was absent from school for three days. When I returned, so did the taunts, especially in that study hall. Though I was very shy at the time, I still found courage somehow to ask them to back off for just one day. I told them my dad died of a heart attack and I just wanted to be left alone.

"Oh your dad died?" one of the demons asked in a sing-song voice. "Oh, I know how he died! He couldn't stand looking at you, fatty. You are so fat and ugly that his heart couldn't take it. Ugh, to see you every day, no wonder he died."

His accomplice laughed and was in complete agreement. They continued to go on about how hard it must have been for my dad to have a fat, ugly child and that he died because of the way I looked. The final blow was when they said my dad died because of me. As usual, the study hall teacher did nothing as tears started to build up in my eyes.

"I see you are going to cry," said the other. "Go ahead fat pig, cry. Cry, cry, cry."

The tears built up but I knew at this point my crying would give them satisfaction, so I held in my tears, grabbed my books, and ran out to cry where none of them could see me - at home.

Names and limitations haunted me throughout my childhood. In school, one student constantly called me a name. He was "proud" of the new word he learned in Spanish class, *isla*, which means "island" in Spanish. He told me I was as big as an island, so my name should be "Isla." I was also called "Fatness." *Hey Fatness! You can't play with us, Fatness!* These along with other names followed me throughout. Through it all, I did not fight back. The advice back in those days was to ignore the insults because it will hurt them if they were ignored. In retrospect, I see this was the worst advice. Ignoring was a challenge, and the bullies continued, determined to make a victim react and "crack."

Gym class was hell for me. Not only was I chosen last for teams (as I highlight in the "Why it Sucks to be Fat" chapter), but I could not keep up. My abilities to run quickly and for longer periods of time were nil. I could not run fast enough to tag anyone in touch football. In tag, I was always "it," the one who had to chase everyone else. I was a slow-moving target, so tagging me to be the one who would be "it" was easy. I could never run fast enough to tag someone else so I was stuck running, unable to catch up with anyone. Children laughed as I struggled to run after them; they were all much faster than me.

No one wanted to include me at all. I was not welcome to join in the games that were played on the playground. Instead, I would walk alone and watch on the side while others played. I used to hate when teachers would ask the class to partner up for a class activity. People avoided me like the plague. There I would stand alone while the rest of the class easily paired. At dances, I had to stand off to the side while guys and girls danced together. No one wanted to dance with me. I was rarely invited to parties or a play time at a child's house after school. In middle school, no one wished to sit with me at lunch. I would find an empty classroom and sit there, eating - alone. In high school, I would either find an empty classroom or sneak out to go home for lunch. Such ways were better than venturing into the cafeteria, only to be told, "You can't sit with us, tubby!"

My weight was also an issue in dancing school. Mom sent me to tap, jazz, ballet and pointe in order to do something extracurricular and to gain some sort of confidence. My first dancing teacher was an amazing person who tried to give me confidence and motivation, regardless of my size. Unfortunately some students in the classes were not so supportive. Some children used to laugh at me when I danced. Some would motion to others and they would snicker. Some would puff out their cheeks, hold out their arms wide, and imitate the steps I would do when we did individual exercises across the floor. Eyes were always on me. Girls turned to each other to whisper, stare at me, and laugh. I was the dancing joke.

Dance recitals were actually fun, but there were some problems. My weight gain during one period of time led me to grow out of one of my dancing school costumes just before the recital. I gained weight between the initial fitting and recital time. A seamstress had to sew in a massive piece of elastic to make the costume fit. Some costumes that I wore over the years did not look flattering. Regardless, the recitals were actually not such a burden, and were actually enjoyable. It was the only time I could feel good about myself. I was up on stage with no one from below to touch me, to say anything. Perhaps some people in the audience said something like, "Look at that fat kid up there," but I did not hear it. Perhaps people laughed, but I did not hear it or see it because the stage was bright and the audience was dark. When dancing on stage, I felt like a shining star. It was the one area on this earth where insults and gestures could not reach me. How I wished for those moments to last longer.

My dieting went full speed ahead in my teenage years. I did the meal shakes for breakfast and lunch. Then, instead of a normal dinner, I would have a burger at a fast food restaurant; so much for healthy eating! Surprisingly, my weight came down and I was starting to look good. Things were going well until I got so sick of having the meal shakes. Once the shakes decreased, my weight increased. That is why I am so against depriving myself of normal foods. It may be easy to stay away from normal foods for a little while, but then the time comes when a person breaks and goes back to the "normal" foods and the same bad eating habits. It is a huge eating bonanza from then on!

After the shake phase, I then migrated to appetite suppressant pills. This did not work for me at all. A vegetarian diet was next. This was not a normal diet of grains, tofu, and such. At the time, I thought a vegetarian diet was just vegetables thrown together on a plate. There was no variety at all in my food choices; I would heat and eat frozen vegetables, which got boring real fast! It got to the point where I was disgusted looking at these wilted, pallid vegetables. There was a great need to try something new.

Frozen diet food was next. Then came the diet food where water is added, and then the "culinary cuisine" is put in the microwave. To put it bluntly, it was freeze - dried astronaut food! It tasted putrid! My willpower and overall dedication to eating right did not last very long on that diet. I gave up and let myself gain weight again.

In retrospect, I see that I rarely put regular exercise into my schedule during these crazy diets. The weight I lost was from food alone. Without exercise, it took much longer to lose the weight. I also had no muscle tone at all. Therefore, I was unhealthy at both higher and even lower weights.

Products from infomercials were my next attempt. I purchased any gimmicky diet plan or exercise tool. I would eagerly use whatever I purchased. The excitement did not last for long. The products were either not as wonderful as advertised, or not wonderful enough to sustain my interest. A small, clunky stepper "machine" was short lived and for a brief time period, became a place to hang my clothes. Some of these items that came with great promise are still in my closet collecting dust.

In my early twenties, I was about ten to fifteen pounds overweight.

My double chin did not yet form. There were lots of flabby, toneless areas. Through it all, getting on and off crazy diets helped me not get overly heavy. I made doubly sure I was on a crazy diet plan so I could lose weight for my wedding. I achieved this weight loss goal and fortunately looked slim at my wedding. Because it was a short term goal and because the diet was crazy, I easily gained back some of the weight I lost. Sadly, those wedding photos of the slim me were used as "ridicule fodder" when a relative on my husband's side verbally noted years later about the weight gain since my wedding:

"Gee, you gained soooo much weight since the wedding," she commented as she gawked at the thin me in my wedding dress. Like a deer caught in the headlights, I froze, doing and saying absolutely nothing about the remark. I was at a loss for words and was heartbroken over such a statement. Though it was true, it did not have to be said; I knew too well I gained a lot of weight since my wedding.

Weighing less helped in the corporate world, since I was on my feet a great deal at the lab bench when I was a scientist. Running around at work had to have helped keep me a bit trim, but I was still overweight. Once corporate travel came into the picture, my leaner self was history. How wonderful and fancy it was for me to have room service, ordering anything I wanted. How amazing it was to travel to my "regular" cities and know which incredible restaurants to go to. Eating luxurious food at the expense of the company was heaven. My travel to these cities was so frequent that the restaurant hosts got to know me! Let the record show that I did not order expensive entrees. I did not order caviar and lobster tail. No surf and turf for me! There was plenty of food that did not cost a lot, but added a lot to my waistline and overall weight. And of course, I made sure I did not waste the company's money and ate every bit of food on my plate. One time I stuffed myself so much that I thought my heart was going to stop!

Many feel that being heavy as an adult would lead to fewer insults. After all, adults are more mature and can hold back comments more than children. Sometimes that is not true; adults could be just as cruel. Some feel an overweight person is lazy. They feel "fat" and "lazy" go hand in hand in. Many make snide comments in the open and aside. One commented that the group should go to a buffet for lunch because by the way I look, it appears that I like to eat a lot! Some honestly feel certain overweight women are pregnant based on the way they are carrying their extra pounds. One man mistook me for a pregnant woman, asking me when I was due. How embarrassing that was. I wanted to crawl in a hole and hide.

Corporate did not seem the best thing for me. I loved the job, but the politics were insane. Some of you thought you heard it all with corporate politics. I am sure I have unique stories. On a daily basis, I was tortured with comments, suggesting that I sit with only higher level people. So much for equal opportunity employers! I was also told that I was too kind to employees who worked for me. Though the work was completed in a timely manner and was of a good quality, upper management did not care. My employees also had a positive spirit, and management wanted to take that away from them. These and other comments made me not want to continue corporate life. It was unrewarding and frustrating. It was disappointing to be criticized and watch the loafers shirk their duties and get promotions as rewards. It was time to find a different career, one that would be more rewarding.

I was tutoring and teaching on the side in the evenings, so I decided to pursue these two and collectively make it a full time job. I taught at a college on Tuesday and Thursday evenings. I taught at a high school during the day, I tutored a few evenings a week. These were dream jobs for me because I loved teaching and helping people overall. I enjoyed what I did. Aside from the enjoyment, another great factor was that being away from corporate travel allowed me to drop a few pounds once again.

Once I had my son, guess what shot up again? You guessed it - my weight. After having my son, I decided to drop the teaching positions. They were not as flexible but tutoring was, so I decided to concentrate solely on my tutoring business. It did give me the flexibility to spend more time with my son. When I returned to tutoring, I found my hours increasing and my business beginning to thrive. I was away from the house during lunch, dinner, or both. Instead of packing a sensible meal, I decided to eat out and treat myself. I had a huge stack of take - out menus for various eateries. Depending where I was in my travels and what meal I was up for, I would select from my tall stack of menus and order the food to go. The food was all ready for me when I arrived, and I "enjoyed" it by wolfing it down in the car as I hurried to my next appointment. This kind of eating also contributed to more pounds. The weight kept on climbing up. I was way into the obese category at this point in time and was far from being simply overweight.

In addition to eating on the road while working, I ate out with my family. This was great to do together, but my choices were far from healthy. I had to have an appetizer, soup, main meal, and dessert. Soups had to be creamy or they were not fulfilling. Sometimes I had a salad with in addition to the aforementioned because the entrée came with salad. That extra creamy, fattening, artery clogging dressing was a necessity for me. Sharing a dessert was out of the question. I had to have my own and the biggest kind they had. The one small benefit was that I got to eat fruit while eating at restaurants. I gave up eating fruit at home. It came to a point where the only time I would eat fruit was when it was a garnish on my entrée or dessert dish. The overeating spiraled out of control.

Throughout it all, I incorporated what my parents taught me - to medicate myself with food. If I had a bad day at work, I would come home at the day's end and reach for chips, chocolate, or whatever I could find that was delectable and fattening. After all, I deserved it; I had a bad day and needed a reward to feel good. If I had problems with a friend or family member, I would reach for food right away. If I had any kind of problem, food was definitely the solution.

Somewhere along the line even more bad habits worked its way into my life. At one point, I was eating ice cream for breakfast! I felt that after lunch, people eat dessert. After dinner, people eat dessert. So, why not have ice cream for dessert after breakfast? Breakfast is a main meal too, isn't it? Some say it is the most important meal of the day! So there I was, dishing out a nice bowl of ice cream for myself after eating a bowl of cereal. Another bad habit was over frequenting the local candy store. This place made its own chocolates, so it was extremely tempting for someone like me. If I decided to buy a pound box of candy for the family as a treat once in awhile (well, perhaps more frequently than "once in awhile"), I would buy an extra half or full pound of candy and pig out on that in the car on the way home. Because I overindulged on candy beforehand, I was able to control myself around the box of candy I presented to my husband and son. It looked like I could control myself by eating a candy or two in front of my family. I would be embarrassed if my husband and son saw me eat most of the candy. If I purchased my own and ate it privately, they would not be able to see how much more I actually ate. I was a glutton who easily devoured a full half pound or pound box of my favorite chocolates. Another food purchase was half a dozen doughnuts that I would eat throughout the day. Upon my purchase, I would make small talk with the doughnut shop employee, confessing that it was for a party. Looking back, I do not think any of the workers over the years could have cared less. Regardless, I had to make up a lie for my guilty indulgences. At buffets, I would have my husband get me thirds and fourths. By my second trip, I knew what I wanted more of and would ask him to get up and get me my favorites. I felt too embarrassed to go up there more than twice. It looked better if a skinnier person went up there anyway.

At one point I used ridiculous reasoning that food can be great medication for what ails me, a nutraceutical if you will. If I had a headache or PMS, chocolate was in order. That chocolate was supposed to be my true cure for headaches and menstrual cramps. I would eat the chocolate, but it never helped my ailment of the day. One would think I would learn that chocolate was not the cure. I was oblivious for years and the same mistake was made over and over. If my throat was sore, salted pretzels were in order. Forget doing something logical like gargling with salt water. Eating lots of pretzels for its salt content was so much "better." Again, my ailment, this time a sore throat, was not cured. A new discomfort resulted which was an overstuffed, sick feeling. Therefore, eating lots of food was my way of self medication, but I never felt better after eating the aforementioned foods. All of these bad habits and misconceptions helped my weight climb even higher.

The shock came when we went to meet family at the beach. My husband took a few surprise photos of me while I was on the beach with my son, trying to fly a kite. He begged to have a few photos of me with family members and I begrudgingly obliged. It was rare to find many photos of myself. I am the one who usually takes the pictures. You would never think that I was even on vacation with my family. There is little to no photo evidence to show that I was there! I would allow for one photo just to prove I was on vacation with my family! But I knew too well that photos revealed the real me that I did not wish to see.

When I saw the pictures of me from that beach day, I was in shock! My face looked like it was stuffed with marshmallows. I was wide and looked huge from front and side views. These pictures my husband took of me were shocking. I looked pregnant and bloated. Our summer vacation photos were also there. At one restaurant we frequented, a server saw me with the camera and was kind enough to volunteer to take a picture of all three of us. That picture was there and it was horrifying. Sure I saw myself in the mirror and knew I was huge. The photos showed me as a larger person, more enormous than the person I saw in myself. This was a huge wakeup call. This was the last straw. I was tired of being obese and having all the problems that come with it. I decided right there that I had to get my life in order and lose weight the right way. No crazy diets - it had to be a completely new, healthy lifestyle. Each day I couldn't stand looking at myself in the mirror. Looking at these pictures was more horrifying. This unhealthy eating had to stop!

Just when I was all ready to tackle a new life, an unexpected setback occurred. I was on my way to pick up my then four year old son from nursery school, when a driver ran through a stop sign and hit my driver's side. There was no time to swerve; he hit me on the side of my car, so I did not see him coming. My knees hit the dashboard, and I felt the instant aching pain. The hit was so intense, that the man's car did a 180 degree spin and hit the back of my car. I looked at my knees. They were pink from the impact and were getting swollen. I was a broken woman and my car was totaled. I was crying and shaking most of the time. The man who hit me asked me if I was okay. I told him I wasn't. In less than five minutes, a police officer came, along with an ambulance.

The emergency room doctor did not think much of my injury and recommended ice and some type of over-the-counter pain relief medication. Unfortunately, the pain did not go away. After grueling acupuncture and other things that were a waste of time and copay, an MRI was done. I had a torn meniscus in each of my knees. Surgery would have to be done, one knee at a time. Each surgery left me walking with a cane for weeks, having limited mobility. During one of the surgeries, the doctor found that my right kneecap had two cracks in it. Knee replacements may be mandatory in the future. The bad news kept piling on, along with my weight. My weight ballooned to a walloping 272 pounds!

My health sunk to an all time low and high. What was low was my health, and what was high was my weight. Walking became such an effort. My knees were hurting me. The accident got me off track and did not allow me to pursue my weight loss goal. I was pretty much immobile, using a cane to make it to short distances. One day I had my leg propped up and looked again at those horrifying photos of pinguid me . That person in the photo was haunting me. My aggrandizement made me boil inside. Collectively, how I looked and felt made me say, "Damn it, I have to do something about it. I can't take it anymore. I can't stand myself anymore!" I felt like a fat old lady. The extra weight made me walk extra slow. I was out of breath climbing stairs or walking in a mall. This made me hate shopping and walking. I couldn't even keep up with my young son. Playing ball with him was very limited, for I would tire easily. Energy was missing and I felt languid all of the time. Looking at myself in the mirror made me disgusted. I had self hate and nausea. I was tired of not being able to find my size in a department store. I was tired of paying a premium for clothes in a mail order catalog because my size fell into the larger, extra cost sizes. After all, it took so much cloth to make my size, so clothing companies had us large ladies pay more for our clothes. All these factors put a lot of pressure on me and I got to the point where I couldn't take this life anymore. I had to do something to change. I had to reach inside myself and find a way to lose the weight without failing. There had to be a way to succeed this time.

The first thing to tackle was the food. I made sure to ask my doctor for calorie/fat intake per day and make sure I ate the right amount in each food group. I budgeted what I would eat for each meal, writing it down. Planning what will be consumed for the entire day is perfect and was one of my key factors which lead to success. It did not take as much time as I thought! I planned my meals carefully, calculating the calories and fat I would have. Reading labels was essential. If I could not get the nutrition information from a product, I would use one of the many guides out there that lists calories, fat, sodium, and such. The internet was also a great tool for such information. I made it a game, making sure not to go over my limit of what I could eat for the day. My doctor gave me guidelines on the amounts of fruits and vegetables I had to have on a daily basis, and I was true to those amounts. The non starchy vegetables like carrots, lettuce, celery, spinach, and onions were my "limitless" foods where I could have as much as I want and not count it towards my daily calories. There were days in which a special event would put me over on required amounts, but I exercised more and got back on track the next day. Everything was balancing out nicely with my food.

Though I knew how much I could eat, a challenge was the portion sizes and honest measuring. Because of my massive eating habits, it was difficult to originally do portion control or even know how much was a "normal" amount. I remember trying to measure out a half a cup of ice cream. There I was, dipping the big spoon into the ice cream, taking two heaping spoons to my mouth before I would put anything in the measuring cup. This occurred similarly with other foods that I was to measure. I was incredibly weak when it came to portion control. I knew measuring would be a challenge, but I was determined to do something about it and eventually get to measuring honestly and accurately. One trick I utilized was measuring ahead of time after I brushed my teeth. This included ice cream! I measured it out in a small bowl and stashed it in the freezer until ready. Sometimes measuring had to be done as the foods were cooked and ready. This was done more honestly because it was not a dessert! The cheating with the measuring occurred mainly for desserts!

What made me fail the most at losing weight were external factors. These made it so difficult to control portions. I thought of the top problems that caused me to overeat: stress, food pushing friends/relatives, parties, restaurants, working and being on the road constantly. I paired each problem with a solution. I tried it out and fine tuned along the way. To take it further, I came up with more challenges and asked friends to share their biggest obstacles that are difficult to overcome. And I came up with tips and tricks for those too! All of these were written down as not to forget and proceeded to follow my own advice!

The next sector to tackle was exercise. I must say that I was proud of how I handled my exercise. I did not try to push myself to long periods of time on the cardio machines, only to find myself quitting. I started at low settings. I remember setting my speed on the treadmill to 2.5 and only being able to do 15 minutes. That short period of time seemed to drag on and I couldn't wait for it to end. The treadmill would get boring from time to time, so I migrated to the elliptical machine. I would then do crunches. I started with 50, which again, was a challenge. As I progressed, time on the cardio machines became easy. I slowly graduated to a setting of 3.5 on the treadmill, going for 30, then 60 minutes. The elliptical was set with resistance, also for 60 minutes. Crunches eventually increased to 600 of various types! To avoid boredom, I incorporated a cardio machine, crunches, and weights. Soon I found myself bench pressing. To spice things up, I would take a class in Pilates, Yoga, Zumba (a kind of dance exercise class), or Spinning. I also invested in a cheap pedometer which was part of an entire different game. I would strive to increase the number of steps I took each day to beat the previous record. Exercise actually became enjoyable and I wanted to do more of it. I saw improvements, and I saw an increase in my social level. I started increasing my days of working out, giving me the opportunity to meet more people.

The pounds came off slowly and steady during this time. I was so proud to lose my first ten pounds but it was also disappointing because people did not notice, not even my husband. I was so huge that ten pounds did not show on me. After about the twenty pound weight loss mark, people were starting to notice. The number of compliments I received during my second year of my lifestyle change and onward were more than the compliments I received during my entire lifetime! My friends noticed the new me. Clients noticed as well. People at my local gym were complimenting me, cheering me on. They alone gave me such a positive spirit. They were validating my efforts and gave me such confidence.

Rewards became endless and they grew. A big milestone was when I went to try on a pair of jeans in the plus size section. It was too large, so I tried on the next smaller size. That too was large. I tried on the smallest size in the plus size section. That also was huge! Thus came my migration to the "regular size" section. I certainly found my size there. This meant a lot to me; I got teary and touched. I was now a "regular" size. No longer would I have to find small pickings of unstylish clothes. I would not have to trudge to the basement of the department stores to find clothes in my size. As long as I kept taking care of myself, I would be a regular size. It was also wonderful to wear jeans again instead of loose elastic slacks.

Clothes rewards continued onward. A new group of stores was open to me; I was able to walk into more clothing stores that had my size. At my heaviest point, I got to learn which shops not to bother walking into. It was clear that my size would not be found there. This time I was able to explore new stores, and could find clothes that would actually fit me. I was never a "fashionista" because it was tough to find clothes I loved. Aside from the fact that finding my size was difficult, sought after styles also looked horrible on me. Having the freedom to choose made me morph into a person who loves clothes. I always hated belts because I looked horrible in them. They were so confining, especially after consuming a huge meal. Now I absolutely love belts! Tank tops used to be appalling to me; now I wear them many times during the summer. Sometimes I wear workout tank tops to the gym. It is amazing what we think we hate. I hated things that I either could not fit into or looked atrocious in. Once I could wear these with pride, I actually enjoyed wearing these articles of clothing.

I started noticing changes in my body. Sure, I could notice that I looked thinner. Certain parts seemed to change quickly, where I noticed something I didn't notice before. My rear end seemed to change overnight! I was showering one day and happened to look back. What I would usually see is a small "table." My butt was so huge that it stuck out. I used to put myself down, thinking it was such a big table, that people can set their drinks down on it. This time, my butt was flat; nothing was sticking out. The double chins seemed to disappear and my face was more chiseled looking. I started feeling my pelvic bones instead of fat. I remember lying on a bed in a hotel room and noticing that a big stomach was not blocking my view directly in front of me. The changes were miraculous!

Soon I became thinner than the people in my life who made snide comments. Life was good, real good. People approached me often, asking me for my "secrets." This was difficult to sum up in a sentence or two. There is no magic pill or special device. It is not just eating right and exercising. It is changing mindset and boosting positive spirit. It is a game plan to handle things that may upset healthy eating. If I had a dollar for every time a person asked me for my tricks, I would be a very rich woman! Clients, gym members, friends, relatives, friends' friends, and the like would all ask. These questions influenced me to write this book. Diet is important - so is exercise. The mind and spirit also need to be conditioned and connected. Additionally, special "tricks" need to be incorporated in life to ensure a continued healthy lifestyle. What I did in great detail to be successful and maintain such success is laid out for you in this book.

It has been a roller coaster with ups and downs. Through the challenges, problems, pressures, and knee surgeries that made me temporarily immobile, I made it through and have been able to maintain. I am now down 125 pounds, surpassing my original 100 pound goal. It is shocking to be a size small after being described as large or extra, extra, extra large!

As you can see, life was not easy for me. Sadly, people's unkind words, treatment, and unfortunate events made me retreat inside myself. I was not outgoing and I had self hatred. Fortunately I was able to take the negatives and make them strengths in the end. I was one of the lucky ones who turned my life around through a lot of hard work and focus. I see a lot of others like me, adults and children alike, retreated and defeated. We do not have to be scarred for life and just leave things the way they are. We can indeed be different people and change our lives for the better. Therefore, if I can do it, you can do it! If I could find the confidence after being pummeled with insults and overall negativity, so can you. I feel worthy and am not that hurt, tortured kid with low self-esteem from years ago. You can get a lot of that confidence too. You can succeed without being born with the "right genes." So no more excuses - go for it! If I can do it, you certainly can!

CHAPTER 2

Why It Sucks To Be Fat

You hear it over and over again. The talk shows, news programs, and articles all mention the detrimental effects of being overweight. To put it bluntly, being fat can increase the chances of diabetes, heart disease, and cancer. Of course more risks can result health wise. What these channels of communication fail to mention are the psychological effects that pile on just like the fat does. They stick to you and are tough to get off. Most people who are overweight do not deprive themselves of food. What results however is deprivation! I thought it would be helpful to list some of my detriments as a result of being overweight. Perhaps you can identify with some. If you are not very overweight, many of these factors are what you have to "look forward to" if you reach obesity. Over the years I would hear the talk about health risks. Unfortunately it did not sink in because I was tired of hearing the same boring public service messages. If I knew about more of these restrictions that result from being overweight, I really do not think I would have let myself go as much. Collectively, these factors made me do something about my weight. Each problem amassed to a separate weight of its own, putting pressure on me in addition to the pressure I felt from my own weight. The emotional downfalls and lack of ability highlighted below can be enough to steer you in a healthier direction.

You Can't Do a Lot of Things

Having extra fat around can weigh a person down. Dragging those extra pounds makes everyday life very difficult. My life of being overweight, and later obese, was challenging for me. There were so many things I either couldn't do, or did with great difficulty. Perhaps some of you, either overweight or obese can already identify with some of these physical challenges.

Going up and down steps was a chore. I would be huffing and puffing as if I ran a marathon. There are stairs in our home, and sometimes I had to walk up and down them quite often, especially if I had forgotten something or if it was a very busy day. If a mall escalator was broken, the stairs were my only option. The extra steps were even more exhausting and I would be extremely out of breath. It was frustrating when I was unable to do what I wanted. There were limitations and difficulties along the way.

Walking in general can be tiring. Long distance walks were extremely trying for my large body. I used to hate shopping of any kind because it involved too much movement and too much standing for me. Walking in a big parking lot to get to a concert was an arduous trek. A day in a theme park would make my knees hurt and I would be absolutely fatigued. Sometimes I would send my husband and son to venture without me while I rested on a bench. They got to enjoy rides and attractions while I sat, alone and miserable. Walking in the sand was extremely challenging and embarrassing. One time we met family on the beach. A group of them decided to take a walk and I, who wanted to be with them, tagged along. Walking in the sand is a tremendous challenge compared to walking on grass or on a standard floor. Everyday walking was taxing, so walking in the sand was even worse! Everyone else in the group moved at a decent pace. I felt I was sinking in the sand as I took each step. Dragging one foot up and advancing it forward felt like I had fifty pound weights attached to each leg. Before I knew it, everyone else was ahead of me and I was lagging behind. I felt so hurt that I couldn't keep up. I felt like a loser. The pain subsided a bit when a family member noticed my struggle and stayed behind to keep me company during my arduous trek in the sand.

Riding a bicycle was almost impossible for me. I felt the wheels sink down as soon as I put my weight on the thing. My area where I live has a lot of hills, so peddling was impossible. Bicycle rides became very short, and I ended up walking my bicycle up these hills. So much for riding to get my exercise! I got frustrated with the bicycle and let it collect dust in the garage.

Certain activities have weight limits. One I can remember well was horseback riding. It was an optional excursion when my husband and I took a cruise to Mexico. The problem was that there was a 200 pound limit. I realized I was well over the limit and could not take advantage of a fun opportunity. The horses were more of the dwarf horses, so these poor things could not support my weight. There was no way I could ride on a horse; I could potentially hurt the poor thing. My weight kept me from an amazing excursion through the countryside.

You Need New Clothes, and That's Not a Good Thing

If you gradually grew larger like me, you had to buy new clothes because you could no longer fit into the old ones. It is so sad to try on a pair of pants and it doesn't fit, especially if they are elastic pants! If the pants just about fit, they are so tight that the fat bulges over. Sometimes the elastic cuts into the waist area. It is painful to remove these pants at the end of the day. It is awful to try on a button down shirt, and see that it is so tight in the front, that the openings between buttons gape open to show my bra. This is definitely humiliating! From experience, it is a fabulous feeling to buy new clothes because of weight loss. However, buying because of a weight gain is depressing. Enthusiasm waned when I had to buy a larger size. I had to change from a size 2X shirt to a size 3X shirt. At that point in time, many stores did not carry size 3X. This forced me to primarily order online. The choices were far from flattering as you will later read.

Instead of trying to lose weight to rectify the problem, I came up with a ridiculous solution. I would buy new clothes in a larger size, but they had to be baggy and/or have elastic. Therefore, if I gained, I could still wear it and not have to purchase new clothes. I'm "proud" to say that I didn't have to buy new clothes until I gained more than thirty pounds. Then I had to go get new clothes. This was a terrible alternative than simply losing a few pounds and keeping my existing clothes.

Paltry Choices, The Dungeon, and the Clown Clothes

It is true that extremely overweight people have a tough time finding their sizes. Unfortunately, many stores do not carry plus sizes. I cannot tell you how many times I walked into a store and saw a blouse or dress shirt I really loved. After searching through several piles, there was no 3X size in sight. Sometimes there was nothing even close to a size 3X! If there was a 3X shirt to be found, it would be the ugliest shirt! The prints were too busy and the buttons were often tacky and huge. I guess some clothing manufacturers believe obese people like to draw attention to themselves, so they think loud clothes are the way to go. It is not enough that the waifs stare and snort when an extremely overweight person walks by. The clothes even draw more attention! I also guess that clothing manufactures believe that large people should wear large buttons. When my size was found, it was usually the same style - clown clothes. The shirts found in my size were mainly loud prints - too loud for my taste. In desperation, sometimes I did purchase these tacky prints. Boy did I look lousy in them! And most of the time the dreaded large buttons were included. If the prints didn't draw attention, the buttons did!

I mention a dungeon in the title because that's where my size would be if a store should carry it. In two stores I shopped at, the plus size clothing would not be located with the "other" clothes. It would not be with the women's clothing next to the "normal" sizes. It would be in the dank, dark basement with bedding and reject items that were sold at a deep discount. The basement area was not as nicely decorated or as "warm" as the other floors. It even smelled damp and the lighting just wasn't the same. I felt punished for being obese. I could not shop in a nice area. The stores might as well have said, "Down to the dungeon, you fat, scurvy knave!"

Your Clothes Cost More Because You Are Fat

Because it was difficult to find clothes in department stores that fit me, I resorted to catalogues and online ordering. Though I was indeed able to find my size this way, it was still humiliating. I know people, both overweight and not, who shop from catalogues without shame. There should not be any shame in shopping this route. However for me, it was shameful. This was my only avenue to get clothes in my size.

What hurt me most while shopping this way was the price. Let's say that the cost of a shirt was $50. That was for sizes XS, S, M, and L. However, sizes that were 1X, 2X, and my size, 3X were sometimes $10 to $15 more. Even when I was a size 1X, before gaining more weight, I had to pay a higher price for the same outfit compared to the price set for the small, medium, and large sizes. I realize it takes more cloth to make a larger person's clothes. However, as an overweight person, the message is more negative. It is as if the clothing manufacturers are directly telling me, "Because you are huge, you have to pay more money for your clothes. As a punishment for being enormous, you have to pay more." Don't we suffer enough?

Sometimes the clown look did not escape me when I ordered from catalogues. One time I ordered a solid blue shirt in size 3X. It arrived with huge white buttons! The shirt did not look like this in the picture! I still had the original catalogue, and paged through it until I found the photo of that very shirt. The buttons were small and blue, not white. I did not get what I paid for. Back it went, and I lost money paying for the shipping to send it back. This could have been avoided if I was able to purchase clothes in an average store.

The Dreaded Carnival/Amusement Park

Going to a carnival or amusement park has a lot of downfalls if you are overweight. Walking around becomes a laborious task. Even standing on long lines to see or ride an attraction becomes a burden as well. It is so tiring for an overweight person to walk or even stand. Additionally, the unhealthy food puts stress on the system. The corn dogs, soda, burgers, chips, ice cream, popcorn, funnel cakes, and other delicacies can weigh a person down. And sometimes I would eat those corn dogs, burgers, chips, ice cream, popcorn, and funnel cakes, all in one day! The enemies that lurk are not only the foods, but the carnival rides. How frustrating it is to stand on a long line for a ride, and then squeeze into a seat that does not quite "fit". Sometimes there were weight restrictions, and I made sure I read the weight limitations that were posted. It would be humiliating to be turned away because of a weight limitation. Sometimes I was afraid that I could not fit on a ride. It would be embarrassing, total degradation.

For me, the dreaded lap bar was my humiliation. This is the bar that pulls down on the rider's lap so he or she will not move forward or upward. Usually the riding compartment seats more than one, so others sit together. When the rider operator pulls down the lap bar, whose stomach is the first to get in the way? Mine, of course! To further the humiliation, the operator tries to push it down further, with little success. My big stomach was stopping the bar from appropriately securing other riders. They were fortunate enough not to fall out although they were loosely secured. I was always sad and humiliated after facing the dreaded lap bar.

Another horror on these rides is the individual seat rides. Some are two and three seat rides. These have individual seats and they are very close together. My butt was big and the fat would pour over my designated space. My waist was bulging with fat and would also spill over into someone else's space. Fortunately that person who would be the victim of space invasion would be my husband. I do thank him for being so patient and accepting, but it was a factor that gnawed at me. Because of my fat spillage, I would try to sit on the end so I could only affect one victim. Unfortunately, riding these attractions does not always work out the way you strategically want. Sometimes another victim, a stranger, would be ordered to sit next to me. How sorry and embarrassed I was, to invade his space and have my fat roll onto him.

One carousel I rode on had a weight restriction. Those weighing 250 pounds and over had to sit on stationary horses that did not move up and down. I was in this 250 pound range and ended up riding in a stationary seat. No up and down horses for me - the poor things could not support my weight.

People Think You Live For Food

A lot of people lack sensitivity. They do not know what a struggle it is to be inside a fat body. Some people thought I was fat because I loved food. Well, I did enjoy what I ate, especially the rich desserts and snacks, but it was not the true reason for being overweight. I was an emotional eater. If I had a problem, a heaping bowl of ice cream was my friend that would temporarily soothe the pain. I didn't know how to eat. At the time, I also hated myself and would tell myself daily that I can never succeed at a diet.

Ignorant people in my life thought lots of food would make me ecstatic. Remember the story mentioned earlier about the buffet? The person who said that we should go to a buffet because it looks like I enjoy eating should be ashamed. True, it was a mean spirited comment, but did he really feel I love to eat more than the next person? For instance, an overweight person will not enjoy ice cream more than a thin person. This is not always the case, yet some feel overweight people are so much more in love with food!

Another coworker saw me eating my lunch. It was something simple like a sandwich. She had to stop and inform me of her "observation."

"Wow, it looks like you are really enjoying your food," she said.

I must admit, I was too stunned for words. I was unprepared for that kind of comment. She smiled and simply walked away. I never watch myself eat in front of a mirror, but I know I am not smiling and rolling my eyes with delight as I take a bite. I do not react like a show host from one of those shopping channels who takes a bite out of a cheesecake or ham he or she is selling. When they take a bite, they close their eyes or even widen them, showing what they are eating is so delicious. I know I ate normally and had a neutral expression like anybody else. I didn't smile as I ate, and certainly didn't show expressions like these show hosts. It was easy to understand - there were prejudices. The person saw me, an obese person eating, so I must be enjoying it because I am fat and love, love, love food.

People at restaurants were not sympathetic either. About 99.9%

of the time, I would clear my plate. After all, I was taught to clear my plate as a child, and this way of thinking continued into my adult life. There would not be one morsel of food left. This led to comments by the wait staff. It would be nice if people did their jobs and simply took the food away. On a number of occasions I would hear, "Wow, you really cleared your plate! You must have really liked your food." Sometimes I would hear "Wow, you finished that so fast! It must have been good." Perhaps I was too sensitive regarding these comments because I had a lot of pounds packed on. But I do think comments like these should be avoided by all servers…just take the food away; no comments are necessary.

Friends (and Enemies) Ridicule You

Words can hurt more than we can understand. Words hurt so much and can lead to much more than hurt feelings. People have killed each other over words, and have even taken their own lives. Unkind words make people feel worthless, especially if the same message is repeated over and over again. I was a chubby kid and children made sure to tease me about it. "Tubby," "Fat Girl," "Loser Lori," and other hurtful labels would be said in my presence. Imagine the names I was called when I wasn't around! Previously mentioned, one called me "Isla," the Spanish word for "island" because I was as big as an island. Two family members would often sing, "I don't want her, you can have her, she's too fat for me." One girl in elementary school called me a fat slob every time she passed me by in the hallway. Other names would incorporate "fat" and a select curse word, which is not worth mentioning here. You can only imagine how bad these names were.

Then there was that famous insult by that family member on my husband's side. She looked at my wedding photo one day when she came to visit. She squinted at it, scrutinizing it. She then said in a sing song voice, "Wow, you gained **so** much weight since you got married."

I felt my face get hot but I bit my tongue, offering no reaction. I wanted to say:

Hmm, gee, I didn't notice. Oh, thank you so, so much for bringing that to my attention. I guess I didn't figure it out when all my old clothes didn't fit me and I had to buy new ones. I thought my husband shrunk my clothes to spite me! All these years I thought he was trying to get even with me for no reason! What a valuable piece of information that just had to be brought to my attention. I was just so oblivious regarding my weight gain! Thanks again for pointing that out to me!

Many reach for the "fat" comment for jokes or for a retort in a debate, just to hurt another. When there is a disagreement, people reach for the lame fat comments instead of focusing on the reasons for dissatisfaction. It is an insult of convenience. For example, in an interview, one celebrity called another a "fat pig." Sure, he is allowed to disagree with another. However, the "fat factor" should not be brought into it. Fat has nothing to do with the matter at hand, yet people reach for it because "fat" and largeness are easy targets. Some reach for the fat comments to get a cheap laugh. An example is during a season of a celebrity dance competition. One of the dancers did a dance that had the judges screaming for more. This celebrity had been struggling with her weight and was doing the best she could. A certain "comedian" commented on her dancing, using pig references for his descriptions. He basically said she was a fat pig, moving her hooves. Most were infuriated with his joke, including the ridiculed celebrity. Another lame part was that the comedian was very overweight years prior, but later lost the weight successfully. One would think he would remember where he "came from." The bottom line is that fat comments are used as weapons for arguments, and for cheap jokes when original ones do not surface in the brain. The fat jokes and insults are the low blows and desperate jokes people should be ashamed of. Therefore it sucks to be fat for these reasons. If there is an argument with a heavy person, weight oftentimes comes out in insults (i.e. fat slob, that fat jerk, the nerve of that fat pig) and the subject at hand is minimal. A heavy person is subject to jokes, whether it be a celebrity, or a person with fiends among business associates, family, and friends.

True, people will have something to say. If it is not about weight, it could be about a facial feature, a personality trait, a lifestyle choice - anything! But it is important to note that people who have a lot of extra pounds are the target of jokes/cruel words both in their presence and absence.

I have encountered many confessions after losing all of my weight. People thought I was ugly and/or pregnant because I was so huge. Some even admitted to ridiculing me when I was out of earshot. Now that I lost the weight, I was beautiful in their eyes. People would confess that they perceived me in a negative way because I was fat, but now I am A-OK with them! This is supposed to be a compliment to me. I am supposed to be impressed. Instead, I accept it, but let such ignorant words roll off my back. I just file these people under "shallow" and watch my back. Here are some of the "beauts" that are so memorable:

"Man, after all these years, you finally look good!"

"I thought you were pregnant for the longest time, but when no baby came, I realized that you were just fat. But now look at you - wow!"

"Hey, who was that fat old woman?" "Look at you now!"

"I didn't know how you could have run after a toddler being as big as you were. Your son must be happy now that you lost weight."

"Wow, you look great. Your husband **now** must find you attractive." (Oh, so did he think I was a fat troll before the weight loss?)

These people mean well, but the "fat, old woman," was still me. Also, there are a lot of people out there who look as I did. Are they unacceptable and ugly too? No way! Therefore, I find such words insulting to me and others who look just as I did.

Sweaty, Embarrassing Spots

I hold nothing back from you. Some things are super embarrassing, but I cannot keep it to myself. These things are true problems that result from having the extra weight. I was never one to sweat, but as I put on more pounds, I smelled and I was sweaty. Sometimes my shirts showed my sweat stains. I even resorted to men's deodorant to fight the sweat. Because my stomach was so incredibly large, it dangled down my legs. It was sweaty in the area where it hung over and made me smell more. To remedy that, I had to put rolled up scented baby wipes underneath my stomach to absorb the sweat and odor. They never fell out - the dangling fat secured them into place. It was a true challenge to make myself look and smell presentable. I was always worrying about my smell.

School Gym Classes Were/Are Hell

Aside from taunting and teasing from fellow classmates, gym class can also be hazardous to an overweight person's well being. The way our gym class ran throughout my entire elementary school years was the captains system. These individuals chosen as captains were always the popular kids. Our gym teacher did not make it a fair system that allowed everyone to get a turn; the popular kids always got to be the captains. I encouraged my mom to call the teacher every few months to give me a chance to be captain. Each captain was free to choose who he or she wanted on the team. The captains took turns, choosing a student to join the teams. Guess who was the last one to be chosen? Yes, it was yours truly. I felt so inferior, like a complete loser. Half the time, the captain would sigh as he or she would choose me, the last student who was not chosen for a team. It was the disappointing, "Oh, well, I guess I am stuck with Lori" sigh. If I was captain as a result of a phone call from Mom, I was then out of the running to be selected. I could be the one who did the choosing for a change. If you are a gym teacher reading this, I urge you to stop this "captains deal" right away. Just divide the class into teams so no one feels like a reject.

Fat Makes You Old

Another of the many things I discovered about fat is that it makes you old. Dozens of people who look at my before pictures say that I looked much older when I had all that weight on me. Losing all of the pounds has made me look ten years younger. After taking a good look, I see they are right. The pudgy face and double chins did indeed age me beyond my true years. Losing this weight helped me not only look young, but feel young. I even started wearing youthful looking clothes and was able to get away with it without looking ridiculous! So start losing weight so you can look and feel younger!

Self Hate Is Possible

If we are not happy with how we look, then how can we be happy with ourselves? We all should be perfectly happy with and love ourselves. Others like me are more hateful with ourselves. When I was overweight, I hated myself. Getting up in the morning and looking in the mirror disgusted me. Putting on a huge shirt and noticing the split side seams angered me. The shirt was huge enough, and I was popping out of it, splitting the seams! If I was out of breath, I cursed myself and my large size. I so hated my size, that I sometimes cut the size tag out of my clothes so I did not have to look at it as a reminder of my failed attempts to lose weight.

Insults to me from me would enter from time to time. For instance, if I was driving and came to a bridge that posted a weight restriction (let's say four tons). I would mutter to myself, "I guess you can't go over that bridge, Lori. That's how much you weigh." There was a letter "F" on my license plate. When I randomly received this plate, I attributed the "F" to stand for "fat" and "failure." As you can see, I was unfair to myself and very unkind. Instead of loving or even liking myself, I was my worst enemy.

You Don't Get to Live Your Life to its Fullest

Let's face it - being overweight weighs people down, so much so, that it prevents people from getting up and living life. Some of us become couch potatoes. Others are so humiliated about their weight that they rarely or never venture out. Sitting in the house and being a recluse is not a way to live life to its fullest. Not being able to move or do can prevent us from an experience. Going out and living life is the best route to take.

For a time I did not want to leave the house. I did not want to go places, especially fancy ones. That would mean I would have to dress up and I was so dissatisfied with the way I looked. I had my husband get take-out food for us instead. When we did go out, it had to be at an eatery where it was okay to wear sweatpants and a baggy shirt.

Because I was very overweight, I could not enjoy certain activities. I was either too large to go on rides or horseback riding trips or I was too tired to follow through with a fun activity. I definitely did not live life to its fullest.

The Media Thinks Overweight People Are Jokes

I have seen the covers of magazines over the years, and many run the major headline: *Celebrity Gains Weight*. Some basically send the message: how dare you walk out of your house when you are fat? You have no right to walk out of your house fat! Now we will take pictures and ridicule you! Oprah has been the victim of this media expose. They show the before picture of the once slim Oprah, and the after picture of the heavier Oprah. This follows by digs and other degrading comments. This always bothered me. It did not give me the pleasure to see celebrities gain weight. Some gained sorrier amounts of weight compared to me, but it did not make me feel better. I looked at the message from another angle. The media is saying that it is not okay to gain weight, and now the overweight celebrity is a joke and is unacceptable. Many of these digs come from beach photos, the perfect opportunity to show more skin, and therefore more flab. The "beached whale" type of comment is almost always included in the caption. If comments were not enough, the magnification of the "flab" was enough to make me boil. I remember poor skinny Princess Diana was on the cover of one of these magazines. Her thigh was magnified in the photo to show "cellulite." How disgusting it was for them to do such a thing. It was highly exaggerated. No wonder Princess Diana was bulimic at one point of her life. Everyone was telling her that she was fat! If she did have cellulite (I personally doubt it), why is that fit to print? That is why I personally ban magazines like this. Any magazine that makes fun of overweight people does not get my support. These magazines are telling you that it is not okay to be fat, and that you are a joke if you are.

You now know why it sucks to be fat. After reading this, don't you want to make that vital change? Don't you want success?

You may be obese like I was. Or you may have only a few pounds to lose. So if you are obese, why stay that way? If you are just a little overweight, why stay that way or work your way to obesity? If you are not happy with yourself, then you must change. You cannot allow things to stay the way they are or have any of the aforementioned problems happen to you. Do not permit excuses to dominate your life. It is high time to do something about it!

Are you ready? Then turn the page and begin the journey of changing your life!

CHAPTER 3

A Short Note...What to do Before Delving into the Suitcase

Many people get a checkup before traveling abroad. Before taking any "journey," whether it be a staycation or somewhere far, a checkup is strongly recommended. This is used for a baseline. If you were like me, you have not cared or even made time for yourself. If you were like me, you would pass on seeing the doctor for years at a time. No need to hear bad news or another lecture about losing some weight. It was frustrating for me to go so it ended up being years since I saw a doctor. Not only did my weight officially categorize me as "obese," but I had high cholesterol to boot. I must say that although it was not great news at the time, it made me much happier to see the difference in my cholesterol and health overall after the 125 pound weight loss. So see where you are at for a baseling and make that difference. As you change your lifestyle and take better care of yourself, be sure to get regular checkups. You will see the progress and ensure you are maintaining.

While you are there, ask your doctor to give you a "budget," the calories and fat you can "spend" each day. Definitely consult your doctor; there may be other factors you must consider such as salt, cholesterol, and/or sugar intake. Also find out dairy, carbohydrate, vegetable, and meat servings you need each day. Once you get your daily "budget," you must then spend it wisely. Below are examples of core dishes you can start with as a base. The calories and fat listed are <u>very</u> approximate. I actually averaged the numbers from various websites to give you an estimate. Oftentimes such nutritional information is found on the product or on the manufacturer's website, which are the most reliable sources. There are also recipes throughout the chapters which are also helpful. Again, ALWAYS consult with your doctor to find out about your nutritional requirements. We are all different and have various needs. Men's nutritional requirements are different from women's. Some are diabetic and have to watch sugar intake. Others have heart or cholesterol issues. Some can tolerate gluten, some have severe food allergies. Let's face it, one standard number of calories, fat, and the like cannot be applied to every person's needs. Also, I am not a nutritionist, nor do I claim to be. My instructional piece comes from how to handle external factors that cause us to overdo it. Get nutritional requirements from your doctor first.

Some people are unsure of portions. You can always check with your doctor to determine the best portions of food per meal. However, here are some examples of decent serving sizes:

- 4 ounces cooked grilled chicken breast (no oil used in cooking) - 160 calories, 3.5 grams fat
- 4 ounces of cooked steak (not cooked in butter or oil) - 180 calories, 9 grams fat
- 1 cup of cooked pasta/ ½ cup sauce/1 tbsp grated parmesan cheese - 200 calories, 6 grams fat
- 1 cup of cooked rice with vegetables - 240 calories, 0.4 grams fat
- 1 cup of low fat vanilla yogurt with ¾ cup strawberries and ½ cup unsweetened shredded wheat - 200 calories, 3.1 grams fat

Also note that this book is packed with recipes, so please read on to find other options! This is just to give you a head start. The object is to eat healthy and stay within the parameters your doctor gives you. My job is to make sure you stick to the plan, handling all obstacles that come your way!

Now I must have a heart-to-heart "talk" with the people who are like the Lori from long ago. The old person I was did not just overeat. Let's just say that person did <u>way</u> too much overeating! The above serving sizes would not be feasible right away. It is like telling a person who eats six slices of pizza for a meal to cut down to a drastic one slice. That will not work and ultimate failure will occur. Cut back little by little and work your way to the four ounce portions or that one slice of pizza per meal. Drastic cuts will lead to drastic failure, so cut back wisely and work towards smaller portion sizes.

I personally was a five slices of pizza kind of girl. I could easily eat these five slices in one sitting and still have a massive dessert. Gradually, I cut back the number of slices. First, I cut back to four slices. This is not healthy still, but healthier than five slices. Finally, I can eat one slice of pizza for a meal and be completely satisfied. My success is not from drastic changes, but from gradual changes.

Another thing I recommend is to take a few "before" pictures, photos of yourself before you fully start your PERMANENT healthy eating journey. If you are like me, few pictures of yourself exist. Take front and side profile shots. You will be glad you did when the weight comes off and the slimmer, healthier you is formed. You can look back and feel proud of your accomplishments.

Now that you have the prep work done, let us learn about what we need to overcome obstacles in and out of the home. That is my specialty. Feel free to use these tips and tricks with any meal plan/ healthy eating plan you are on. Now photocopy/copy the Notes of Success and Traveling Game Plan located at the end of this book and have it ready to write down tips and tricks!

Core Luggage
Bring With You Everywhere!

CHAPTER 4

Do Not Avoid Your Favorite Foods

Don't you like this book already? I am not one of *those* people who will tell you not to ever eat your favorite foods again. For some, it is impossible to say goodbye forever to foods such as bread. Many diet "plans" involve elimination of certain products. This includes popular foods such as breads and pastas. Some require elimination of certain ingredients such as sugar or flour. I do not personally agree with this. Completely eliminating favorite foods and ingredients like these is almost a sure way to fail. Compliance may last a short or long period of time. In the end, the result is the same. We give up depriving ourselves of these foods and ingredients and return to our old, unhealthy ways. We finally cave in and return to our old bad habits.

This chapter should be held in our core luggage. When a decision to give up a food or foods is made, it pertains to inside and outside the home. Many choose to give up certain foods for a time being, and will refuse to eat it at home, work, party, or restaurant. Giving up certain foods is a challenge that is ephemeral. I was one to give up a food or ingredient, only to go back to it later, eating it in mass quantities to make up for lost time.

Can I live without bread? Absolutely not! I use it for a variety of healthy sandwiches. I eat hamburgers or veggie burgers with the bun. I love eating stuffing on Thanksgiving! I will also splurge and have a roll when dining out. These are all some forms of bread that are a part of my eating life. I also cannot do without pasta. I will have it as a main course or as a side in a variety of tasty ways. Do not expect me to give up pizza. I cannot sit idly by while my family enjoys that amazing food. So if I was to incorporate a no pasta/bread/pizza stipulation into my diet, I would surely fail. Even if I would be able to pull it off at the beginning, efforts would quickly dwindle and I would be back to eating anything and everything.

One can say that carbohydrates are bad and the breads, pasta, and pizza can make people fat. There are two main facts. The first on is that the body needs carbohydrates. The second fact is that we can get fat by eating a lot of almost anything! I will not eat a heaping pile of pasta, but will have a cup of it. Eating two or more slices of pizza is not the best for my diet, but I will eat one slice (see the Pizza Palooza chapter). The frequency of eating pizza is once a month, not every day or even every week. And I can have these foods in moderation and be satisfied with my eating.

Pizza, pasta, and bread are just a few examples of foods that are eliminated for dieting purposes. For others, it can be foods like fries, hamburgers, meat, cakes, and cookies. Some decide to eliminate gluten. Do not confuse favorite foods with those we can live without. For instance, I used to love funnel cakes and zeppoles. I enjoyed them but even in my obese years, I could have lived without them. Now that I changed to healthier eating, those dough based foods submerged in oil would probably not agree with me like they used to. Certain foods that agreed with me during the obese years now make me very ill. It is my lifestyle change to healthier food. My stomach can no longer handle the greasy foods. Though funnel cakes and zeppoles taste great, I can personally eliminate them from my diet.

Enjoy that thick, delicious salad dressing, just not so much of it! A trick I use to get "more" for less is <u>slightly</u> diluting a thick dressing with water. This gives the dressing more spreadability. More salad components would be covered in it. Thick dressings tend to stay in one glob, so we put on more to coat more of the salad. But when we put on more dressing, it helps us put on more weight. Another trick is to dip a fork in a tablespoon of thick dressing, then stab the fork into the salad. The fork is coated with the dressing and does not have too much on it. The dressing gets to last longer and a salad can be coated more with it. Regardless of the trick I use, I would much rather have a tablespoon of fattening dressing than four tablespoons of a diet dressing that tastes rancid. (More about salads in the *Salad Sense* chapter.)

We <u>can</u> eat our favorite foods, just not so much of it. We have to work it into our diet. If we sacrifice our favorite foods in order to lose weight, we are sure to fail. So do not deprive yourself, or else failure is imminent.

CHAPTER 5

Approach With An Open Mind

The next few chapters work on the mind before we get to the body. I dislike diet books that simply tell you what to eat. There is more to weight loss success than the food. Success does not solely lie with eating right and exercising. The mind has to be worked on as well. So to start, we must work on our minds whether in or out of the home.

In order to reach simple and complex goals, something must change. An example can be seen with my tutoring. Though my tutoring business varies, the most sought out tutoring involves preparation for standardized tests. This chiefly involves tests for college admissions. I teach "tricks," to help students get a better score. Some become lazy and do not do such tricks. The primary excuse is that they claim to do the tricks in their head. The second most common excuse is that it takes too much effort to do extra things on the standardized tests. These and other excuses make the efforts moot. They refuse to change and keep taking the test the same way. I tell them that if they do not bring anything new to the "table," then they will not improve their scores. In order to get results, something has to change. The same strategy can be applied to losing weight. If you keep doing the same things and have the same mindset, there is no way you will succeed.

In order to have any chance at success, modifications must be made. We have to think differently and be willing to change our lives. Sometimes we get too comfortable and become conservative people, enjoying things just the way they are. There is no room for change, and we are more comfortable leaving things be. If we do not change, our bodies will not change. They will be the same overweight size or even heavier. If we have that weighed down feeling, we will always have that if we sit idle and let bad habits and bad eating continue.

Therefore, be willing to change and try new things. Remember to take notes as you read this book, writing down things that you need to do differently. Do not think you will memorize everything, so writing things down is essential. Have an open mind to changing your life. Approach this new way of thinking and doing. Approach it with great enthusiasm. More on that in the next chapter...

CHAPTER 6

Grow A Positive Spirit Not to be Trampled On

One of the main things that "killed" my chances of success in losing weight was my lack of positive spirit. I had such evil thoughts about myself that were entering my consciousness on a regular basis. Many of these stemmed from my own creation, but also from the cruel words of the past. I was my own worst enemy. I used to torture myself, degrade myself, and say I could not succeed. My "voices" in my head told me that I will never have self control in or out of the home. After all, efforts were made and failures were the results of such efforts. These degradations made me unsuccessful, and I quit trying to lose weight. I returned to my old ways and just chalked it up to another failure, another thing I cannot do.

When I would have a setback and would eat more than I should have, I punished myself with cruel words. I would say horrible things:

"Lori, you couldn't even control yourself. You ate like a pig, what a loser you are."

"You failed at diets before, so what makes you think you can succeed now? You just proved that you can't do this. This try is no different from your countless other failed attempts."

"Look what you did. You couldn't stick to a diet. You are such an idiot!"

More mental lashings followed when articles of clothing became tight on me. When I tired out easily due to my weight, I resented myself and also shot insults in my mind. It was a hate relationship! I hated myself so much, that I used to tease and insult myself. You read about my insult to myself when I read the weight limits on bridges. When I could not find clothes in my size at a particular store, I used to shoot an insult to myself in my mind: "See, they don't make clothes for those who are the size of a horse or cow. These clothes do not come in huge horsey sizes!" It doesn't matter who my worst enemy is - I hated myself even more than that person!

You may find this surprising, but I do not treat myself like that anymore. I realized that aside from eating poorly and exercising little, my lack of positive spirit was also contributing to my large size and poor health. If I hated myself, there would be no way I could succeed. Why try hard for someone who you hate so much? I had to start liking myself or else there would be no way I could lose weight and keep it off.

If I overeat for a day, and believe me, I do from time to time, I forgive myself. I realize I am human. Sometimes I will let myself go and "live it up." The only time I feel bad is when I physically feel ill from eating rich foods. My body is not used to certain unhealthy foods, and I pay a price when I eat them. This of course makes me eat them less frequently. If I deviate from eating right, I forgive myself and move on. I make sure I am "good" the next day, sticking to my healthy lifestyle.

I had to clear those negative thoughts from my head. I pictured them as evil people trying to rile me up and feel bad about myself. If a negative thought entered, I pictured a big broom sweeping them away, even hitting them to make them scramble. I would not allow the negative thoughts to be completed. I was mindful of them and got rid of them as soon as I was aware of their presence.

There are several books that help people maintain a positive spirit and even drop excuses. I have a few favorites, but with books like these, the "chemistry" between you and the book is important. I would research self-help books on the internet that motivate. These are books that improve a positive spirit. Once you find a few books, go to your local bookstore and page through them to see if they pique your interest. Books like these raise spirits, happiness, and efforts, as long as there is an open mind of the reader. Do try to incorporate self-help books into your reading to build and maintain a positive spirit. It will help strengthen you to achieve goals and to also be a new and improved person! Another important thing to do is tell yourself that you can succeed. Do not allow the negative voices to tell you that failure is all that will be experienced.

When I bowl, oftentimes I would face the chance of making a spare. When I would see the lone pin or a couple of pins left, the old me would tell myself that I will not make the spare. And you know what? I would not make the spare most of the time because I told myself how it was going to be. Once I cultivated a positive spirit, and when faced with that spare, I told myself that I can make the spare...and I did! Most of the time, when I think of encouraging words, I can succeed at what I am doing. If you send positive messages to yourself, the same great results can happen in your life.

Another way to grow a positive spirit is to allow positive comments to come your way. Some of my friends will debate me if I give them a compliment. I could say that the dress is nice, and a friend will challenge my statement, telling me it is not. I could tell someone they look beautiful, and that person will say it is not true. I too was guilty of this. Allow positive comments to come your way. Do not filter or challenge them. Receive such kind words with ease and happiness!

One thing I did to absorb and retain such good words was to

write them on a post-it. When someone gave me a compliment, I wrote the statement on a post-it and placed it on the rim of my bedroom mirror. During my weight loss journey, many remarked how much thinner I what amazing work I am doing in order to be thin. That was on a post-it as well. After waking up in the morning, I look at myself in the mirror and see my reflection surrounded by all these positive messages. It was a sea of positive messages, just for me! Keep in mind that your reflection should not be the only image to be surrounded by the positive messages! Love yourself!

Now that I am getting you on the positive track, I have to warn you about your nemeses, the negative people. Many are sure to damper a day, a belief, or goal. Negative words can stop anyone's dream. We all need to overcome the poison that these pests dish out. It is tough to achieve and maintain a positive attitude. Negativity from one's inner self is tough enough to handle. Horrible thoughts penetrate, which lead to self - hate, overall worthlessness, and thoughts of quitting. As mentioned previously, we need to control these kinds of thoughts and have fighting spirits. What we cannot control are negative comments from the outside world. These pessimists are crass and ruthlessly criticize efforts. It makes it increasingly difficult to have negative people around who criticize efforts. For some, perhaps this is nonexistent. However, the world is teeming with pessimists, many making their ways into our lives. It is important to handle these people appropriately, or else they can contribute to the downfall of your efforts. They do destroy the foundation of your good work, whether they purposely aim to do so or not. We can train ourselves to stop thinking negatively, but we cannot train others to stop dishing out idiotic comments. An alternate way is to filter out the blather.

Here are some traditional comments I have heard over the years:

- *The amount of food you are eating is ridiculous. Is <u>that</u> all you are going to eat?*
- *Why try? You are just going to gain it back anyway.*
- *Isn't that healthier food expensive?*
- *You're only eating that? You'll be hungry in a little while.*
- *How can you eat that? It's rabbit food!*
- *You are big boned. You'll never look thin.*
- *Overweight people run in our family. There is no way you can lose the weight. You are genetically destined to be overweight.*
- *You're no fun anymore.*(This is told to me when I refuse to chow down alongside the negative culprit.)

The comment that hurt a great deal came from a toxic individual who worked out at the gym I used to frequent. This one lacked charm and decency. For his amusement, he enjoyed goofing on people by slinging insults. I personally hate these kinds of jokesters. They basically tell you that you are inferior, and then say, "I was only kidding!" After losing 102 pounds at the time, this dolt had the gall to tell me that it looks like I eat a lot of chocolates. He was telling me in a roundabout way that I was still fat!

After years of hard work, I certainly did not want to hear that I was still fat. Without exaggeration, hundreds of people were telling me how good I look. Gym members, my son's school community, clients, and friends all complimented me on my figure. My own doctor told me that my weight was within normal range and that I did not need to lose more. Now this poison was trying to seep into my pure, positive life and contaminate it with his comment.

At first, I was livid and walked away. The old me would have reached for the chocolate chip cookies to soothe my soul. I was very sensitive to insults, taking them in, internalizing them. After realizing this guy is a bitter, jealous loser, I moved on, maintaining my healthy lifestyle focus. I made sure to avoid him at all costs. I would give a polite wave, then move on to my workout. There was no time for small talk when there is a loser who has diarrhea of the mouth. I only had time for a wave, and no time for his nonsensical words.

Some pessimistic poison people (the PPP group as I "affectionately call them") ridicule my techniques. Some find it odd that I eat with a shrimp fork and baby spoon. Some think I am insane to eat a hamburger with half a bun. I do happen to have a stock answer for those people who make me look like I am doing something wrong:

"Well, doing this doesn't bother me, so it should not be any concern of yours. If it doesn't bother me, then it shouldn't bother you." Most do shut their pessimistic mouths after that comment. Those who continue on with the badgering are more ignorant that the ones who shut their mouths earlier on.

The "sticks and stones" saying is untrue. Names can indeed hurt; words can hurt more than the "slings and arrows" of life that we experience. Words have caused low self esteem, bitter feelings, suicides, and more. Words do cause damage and do prohibit us from accomplishing our goals. Though it is hard to do, we must take in the good words and filter out the bad ones.

Underlings taunted me as a child. They did this to feel better, to feel superior. I absorbed these words and let my soul rot. I was within myself, refraining from reaching out and being outgoing. Self hate developed and I had no ambition. I never fought back to put these miscreants in their places. When I got older and thankfully wiser, I realized the various reasons for cruelty. Here are some reasons that can be applied to those who offer negative comments to you, especially regarding weight loss:

- jealousy
- They are pessimistic by nature. No matter what you do is unacceptable to them.
- An overweight friend/relative does not want you to succeed because he or she will be alone as an unfit person. Misery does indeed love company.
- The person is teased/taunted, and needs to pick on someone to blow off steam. Those who are picked on find pleasure in torturing others.
- Bad times make people bitter. They lost the "rose colored glasses" and can only see things from a negative perspective.
- The individual persona consists of sarcasm and jokes. The person likes to give "ribbings."

Recognize the reasons for the comments, but do not internalize such statements. Recognize the comment as negative or poisonous and file each in the garbage! I personally should have trashed unkind words at a young age, but I did not know any better. And know these cretins are not the experts in "loserology," so do not take their words to be from knowledgeable souls. Always push forward, regardless of what is said. Do not use their negative comments as excuses for grabbing for the sweets. If these people are collectively your roadblock to good health and overall happiness, do not be afraid to let them go. Cut them out of your life, or even drastically reduce your interaction time with them, whether they are a friend or relative. If there is no support, there is no value in keeping that person in your life.

An old friend of mine told me I looked great. "That's wonderful that you lost so much weight, Lori," the old friend said. "But I got to tell ya, if you put that weight back on, I'll walk." I asked my friend if that was a joke. I wanted to confirm the meaning so I could project the right reaction. My so called "pal" said it was serious, and that there was no excuse to gain the weight back. This was opposite of the negativity I have experienced. People usually criticize my efforts; this individual was foolish enough to threaten a loss of friendship if I deviated from my thinner persona. Though it was tough, I cut the friend loose. There was no need for shallow people in my life. If gaining weight leads to the loss of friendship, then that friend can keep on walking.

It is common sense to say that we should ignore negative comments, but do we truly do that? Honestly, no. We cannot help overhearing such garbage, but we do not have to internalize comments and allow such nonsense to affect us in terrible ways. In order to get rid of the negative comments, sweep them out and away from your life. If certain people have to be swept away with the rubbish, so be it. They are obstacles we do not need in our lives.

CHAPTER 7

Push Away the Food Pushers

We have to battle the internal negative spirits, but we must also fight the external ones. Most of us have these "demons" in our lives. These are food pushers. Some have good intentions, some do not. These could be moms who worry about their grown children not eating. Some moms enforce bad habits which they do not realize are wrong, such as eating everything off of one's plate no matter how full one feels. It could be an overweight or not so overweight friend who eats poorly and wants an "accomplice" in her food crimes. It could be a party host who wants you to try a little of this, and a little of that, so you can enjoy the fruits of her labor. Let us not forget the special relative who has to get you to try that homemade dish of fattening food. There are also those who will make that special fattening food that they know you like and must absolutely have upon each visit. These food pushers add to your list of excuses as to why you cannot succeed in a healthy lifestyle. They are always there to get you to eat the wrong foods, and lots of them.

There is only one solution - reject the food pushers! The only problem is that many will be highly insulted. After all, they worked hard making special foods you like. Then you go and reject their offering! The reasons for their hurt feelings will vary and some will be more offended than others. Sadly, there is no universal solution or statement to help resolve all conflicts, but I have a few lines that I use for various people. You will have to use your best judgment, based on personality type, to know which would work with a particular food pusher. Here are some examples:

- *I'll take a little taste, but then I have to be good. Thanks so much for thinking of me.*
- *I would love to, but I ate a lot yesterday and have to be on my best eating behavior today.*
- *Thanks anyway, but my stomach isn't right today. It is a little funny, so I can only eat a little bit (or say that you cannot eat anything at all).*
- *Can we pick a place like _____? (a restaurant that serves healthier food than what the other person/people suggested) I can find better choices for me there.*
- *I know I didn't eat a lot, but you know I love you!*

Pushing away the food pushers will give you more freedom. This will also help stick to your healthy eating plan without having these interferences.

CHAPTER 8

To Drop the Pounds, Drop the Excuses and Lies

There are other things we must drop besides the pounds - the excuses and lies. We do not realize how much they dominate our lives. Such statements we tell ourselves give us several reasons not to try, to not lose weight. They allow us to be the same while we yearn to change deep down inside. They validate our reasons for being overweight and grant us permission to continue life this way. The bottom line is that excuses and lies are crippling and only lead to failure.

First let us tackle the excuses. Here are some common excuses I have used over the years and have heard from others:

- *It's too hard to lose weight. There is no way to succeed.*
- *"Fat" runs in my family. I am destined for "fatness." I have the fat gene.*
- *I failed before, so there is no way I'll succeed this time.*
- *There is too much stress in my life to diet properly.*
- *I do not have the time to exercise.*
- *I do not have the time to diet.*
- *I can't change. The way I am is the way I am.*

- *I just can't control myself at parties/friends' homes/restaurants.*
- *Ice cream (or whatever your favorite food is) is my favorite and I can't stop eating it at all.*

I am sure you can contribute more excuses to the list. The possibilities are endless! Excuses do nothing but cripple us. We remain unhealthy and sometimes deteriorate as the months/years progress. We need to counter the excuses with reality. I will go through all of my excuses and tell you the things I did and how I convinced myself that changing my life is doable.

It's too hard to lose weight. There is no way to succeed.

Life isn't easy. Losing weight is not a simple task. Should we run away and not try because it is too hard? There will be challenges along the way, but we can tackle them one challenge at a time. There may be slip ups from time to time, but that should not lead to quitting!

"Fat" runs in my family. I am destined for "fatness." I have the fat gene.

This is an old tale we tell ourselves. The inheriting of the bad parts even branches out further than weight. People have told me that they didn't get the "math gene." This made them comfortable in doing poorly in math subjects because it was somehow in their destinies. Some say they inherited the literary gene from their mom or their dad. Therefore, academic genes seem to be in existence, because so many people attribute their talents or lack of talents to the infamous intelligence gene. The same goes for the weight gene. People doom themselves from the start. If a relative is overweight, then there is no way to be slim. If people come from a family that primarily has overweight people, they feel there is no hope in losing weight. I had a mix in my family; some were overweight, some were not. Regardless of the tally, I told myself that I have to press forward, regardless of any kind of family history. Just because someone in my family looks a certain way does not mean that I have to be that way as well. Fat does not have to be my destiny and it does not have to be yours.

I failed before, so there is no way I'll succeed this time.

Failures while trying to lose weight are from wrong strategy and from the ease of giving up. Reflect on what made you give up. Did you get sick of the protein shakes and protein bars? My problem was eating diet food. I got so sick of these foods, which I eventually gave up and turned to my old bad eating habits again. I did not know what to eat and how to eat right. I also did not know how to handle myself while at parties or while on business trips. Not knowing what to do and making wrong choices always led to a failure. To make things work for myself, I had to reexamine the mistakes I made. There had to be modifications. After making such changes, I was successful. This time, I lost the weight the right way, kept it off, inspired others, and enjoyed the fruits of my labor! There is no way to succeed if no one sets forth the effort. Successes come from reexamining the failures along the way and fine tuning for success.

There is too much stress in my life to diet properly.

We all handle stress so differently. As a child, we would lash out or overreact. We had to learn to control ourselves. That is what we have to do as adults. We have to learn not to medicate ourselves with food if we are going through tough times. We have to adjust the way we respond to stress. Grabbing for food is not a solution. We cannot use problems as excuses to fail. I convinced myself that the box of chocolates will not solve my problem and I will end up feeling worse instead of better. Stress is not making us overeat, WE are making ourselves overeat, using stress as the trigger. Remember, we all have problems, but food is not always the solution.

I do not have the time to exercise.

This excuse is the most pathetic. We have time to help our family, don't we? We have time for our friends. We have time to do our jobs and make work deadlines. We have time to watch our favorite show. We can even go out to the movies. We have time to chat with others and play around with the computer. Why don't we carve out time for a little bit of exercise? I try to do my exercise in the morning, right after dropping off my son at school. I get it over with in the morning and then have time to do my errands and go to work. I am trying to help my husband exercise, so we do abdominals ten minutes before we go to bed. Although I exercise in the morning, I work out with him so he has the motivation to do it. I have time to go to the gym five days a week, and I work 50 to 60 hours a week, seven days a week. I have a son, husband, and friends to juggle. I used to do volunteer work at an assisted living center about twice a month. I would run a little science presentation for a Kindergarten group in my community to get them excited about science. I am trying to get medical care for a dear friend who does not have medical coverage. Sometimes I have only twenty minutes to duck into the gym and exercise, and due to this limited time, I end up exercising in my street clothes! While everyone is in workout clothes, I am in jeans or shorts, working out. There is no shame and the important factor is getting the exercise in, even though it is for a few minutes. I am just as busy as the next person, yet I make the time for my health. You can work it in, even while waiting on the phone or on a line, or even in a doctor's office. Find the chapter on losing weight while you wait; it is in this suitcase. It gives some nifty ways to work in exercise while we do our everyday "waiting."

I do not have the time to diet.

This is such a lame excuse of mine. I had the extra time to stuff my face with more food, yet I did not have time to eat right. See details from the above excuse. They are certainly applicable to this excuse. We do have time for other things. Why not make time for ourselves? We certainly deserve some time. If we do not make the time, how good are we to anyone else if we get sick or even die due to unhealthy eating?

I can't change. The way I am is the way I am.

I can be the poster child who refutes this excuse. For over thirty years, I never changed my eating habits. I ate when I was sad, I ate when I was happy. I ate when I was stressed. I couldn't measure out small portions. I would eat two heaping spoons of ice cream before I would measure out a half a cup! I ate a full course meal at a restaurant, choosing the creamiest, most fattening entrees on the menu. I did a complete 180 degree turn and do not turn to food for emotional support. I measure things honestly and order wisely. We CAN reprogram ourselves if we allow it and not use an excuse to tell us something otherwise. Anyone can change, no matter what the age. And do not believe the "you can't teach a dog new tricks" saying. Anyone can learn something new.

I just can't control myself at parties/friends' homes/restaurants.

Because I told myself I couldn't do something, I simply did not fight it. If I assigned my weakness, I lived it. If I said I couldn't control my eating at parties, I was right and that was that. I had to think of strategies to handle myself better at gatherings or restaurants. In upcoming chapters, I will give you great tips on how to dine out the smart way. I will also give you ways to handle yourself at parties. It can be done. If I can control myself, then you can too!

Ice cream (or whatever your favorite food is) is my favorite and I can't stop eating it at all.

No one told me that eating right meant that I had to give up all of my favorite foods. I know if I had to give up my favorite foods, I would have to give up on changing my healthy eating lifestyle. We do not have to give up our favorite foods, but we sure have to eat them in moderation. I have a chapter dedicated to eating desserts the right way. If ice cream is your favorite food, you can still eat it in smaller portions and still be satisfied.

A "bonus" excuse I recently heard was the following:

It just won't work.

This was the actual response a friend of mine relayed to me. She has an obese friend and proudly mentioned me and my accomplishments.

"You should talk to her," my friend urged. "She lost so much weight, so ask what worked for her. Maybe she can help you."

"Oh, it just won't work," she quickly said.

"But maybe it will work, you don't even know what she did. Wouldn't it help to at least listen to what she suggests?"

"No, it just won't work."

Again, this is an excuse to justify her present being, to make it okay for her to be in that unhealthy shape. This also validates her decision to do nothing. After all, it just "won't work." She did not even know how I lost the weight. Perhaps it was a doable plan that could work for her lifestyle. Before hearing the plan, she decided ahead of time that it would not work. Why bother? It is obvious to see that certain crazy diets won't work, especially if the diet is so limited. However, rejecting everything is ludicrous.

Once again, I am confident that you can think of more excuses to add to my list of common ones. Regardless of the excuses, you need to break free from them. Do not accept them; if you accept excuses, then you accept failure. Wash away excuses and look towards winning, not losing.

Once you cleanse yourself of excuses, cleanse yourself of lies you will tell yourself. Believe it or not, we do lie to ourselves from time to time and this makes it difficult to stick to a healthy eating lifestyle. The common lie is that we did everything right on a particular day and did not lose weight. More often that is not true. We all sneak in a few goodies that we should not have had. Those few goodies are enough to hamper results. We try to ignore them, thinking that they do not "count."

Not only do we fool ourselves, we try to fool others. Usually we are more aware of the "lies" we tell others. I used to go to various weight loss centers throughout the years where I had to face the scale every week. If there was no weight loss or even a weight gain that week, I would pretend to act puzzled.

"Gee, I don't know what happened," I would say with such drama, as if I was the victim. I would tell the person weighing me in that I was oh, so good all that week, eating right, exercising right, et cetera. In the meantime, I had the images of me eating out three times that week and having a mean "munchee attack" the day before, eating as many unhealthy foods as I could until I felt overly full. And yet I was "surprised" that I did not lose weight. I knew too well why the scale read the number it did. I was honest with myself, yet I put on a performance that deserved an acting award of some sort. If not portraying the victim, I made excuses about it being a "bad week" because it was either "crazy/busy" or stressful. Regardless, I was justifying my inability to eat properly for that given week and giving myself a way out.

Some people lie to themselves so much that they actually believe the lies they divulge. A colleague of mine used to rant about the Weight Watchers diet and said it did not work for her. She said she was doing everything right and was getting no results. Her constant complaining led me to watch her eating habits a little more closely. While she was still on the program, she always purchased breakfast from the cafeteria. On her tray was a toasted bagel with butter. The butter is fattening, and there was a lot of it, but that was not all. She had a tall yogurt parfait topped with a generous amount of granola. A corn muffin also sat on her tray. There was a plate of hash browns and a large cup of orange juice. This was obviously not healthy eating. She was using the points system that was used back then and is still used to this day. She would have had to use the special Weight Watchers book (since there were no nutrition labels on this cafeteria food) that lists items and their point values. It was clear that she was not doing this. I could almost bet that the total amount of calories and fat she was to have in one day was sitting on her breakfast tray alone. Was she doing everything right? Absolutely not! That colleague of mine was kidding herself. She did not follow the plan as she had claimed. In fact, she was eating everything wrong, and eating too many of these "wrong" foods. After this observation, she continued to tell me weeks later that she is still trying but the diet just doesn't work. It cannot work if she is lying to herself.

If we refuse to recognize the erring of our ways, then how can we expect to succeed in weight loss? We have to admit that we "cheated" ourselves with more food. In turn, we have to admit that we need to come up with a game plan so the behavior is not often repeated. This book has a few suggestions based on many of these situations, so please read on and on...

CHAPTER 9

Don't Put Off Losing Weight- Do it Today

To build on the excuses chapter, do not further your excuses by setting a starting date for changing your life. I can't tell you how many times I had to declare a starting date for one of my future failing diets. Since I pigged out that day, I should continue overeating because today is shot anyway. I can start fresh the next day. Well, instead of gaining five pounds from pigging out, perhaps stopping right then and there would only put on two pounds for that day. It is well worth it to take immediate action.

I as well as others make other kinds of starting time excuses. We'll start the beginning of next week, or we'll begin the first of the next month. There is also the popular excuse to wait because it will be a stressful month with what is going on in the family or at work. Most popular is starting the beginning of a new year. Why do you think diet commercials and gym advertisements pop up the end of December through the beginning of January? It is because so many people make that pledge, that New Year's resolution to eat right. It is important to note that another peak time for these ads is summertime. So many of us want to look nice in that bathing suit or that special pair of shorts. The problem is that the time to reach that goal is unrealistic. Most likely it takes months to get results; by then the summer is long gone along with its wardrobe.

The beginning of the year is depressing. Not only are the major holidays over and done with, but the special sales are advertised with such vigor. There are the diet programs, protein bars, and pills. Gym advertisements and exercise equipment commercials invade our television and radio programs. Stores have these kinds of products right by the entrance to remind you of the popular New Year's resolution to lose weight. To see people jump at the chance is sickening. You know they are going to spend a lot of money and see no results, no long term results whatsoever.

At the beginning of January, I see a huge influx of people working out at the gym. By March, it is calm once again. People cannot stick to it. The problem is that the pledge is not so sincere or heartfelt. There is no true determination to do something life changing. It is all based on timing. Therefore, do not wait until the first of the year. To make a pledge because of timing will lead to failure. Make a pledge immediately so you can, without further ado, change your life. Do not wait until the new year, the new month, or even the new week. Start your new life today! If you overate for half of the day, eat right the rest of the day. Be more careful in what you eat and avoid high fat foods.

CHAPTER 10

Avoid Short Term Goals and Take it Slow!

Most of us have done this. We have a big event and just have to lose some weight to look good. Friends just had to lose weight so they could look good in their wedding dresses. Some needed to tone so they could look fabulous in the bikini while on vacation. Others had to lose weight to look good for a family reunion or high school reunion. A friend of mine who is a personal trainer told me he has helped many people lose weight for a big marathon or race of some sort. When the marathon was over, so were their desires to remain fit. Regardless of the purpose, these short term goals turn up empty. Half of the people succeed and do fit nicely into that special outfit for that special day/trip. When the big event is over, they let themselves go and it is back to unhealthy eating and gaining weight. The other half never reach goals and self hatred seeps in. Failure to reach goals is either from lack of willpower or ridiculous aspirations. The first reason is self explanatory; it is easy to lose willpower. The ridiculousness of the goals themselves easily set people up for failure. A common ludicrous goal is to start working out in June to look great for the summer season. It takes a few weeks to see results. Even if a person is successful, true results often do not show up until after the summer season. Therefore, people fail and do not reach their goal date.

Another problem with short term goals is that clear, concise, sensible "game plans" are almost nonexistent. People run for the quickie diet and/or device that will help for weight loss in a hurry. People's goals become unreasonable and approaches are just as ridiculous. Most of the time, people do not reach their goals.

I must admit that I had my own share of failures, or short successes, then fast failures. Sometimes my goals were not attained. I tried to lose weight for my then ten year high school reunion. My weight loss goals were not reached; I was not even close. This failure made me sit home instead of attending the reunion. I did succeed losing weight for my wedding and looked fabulous. Once the wedding was over, I went back to my old eating habits. From the honeymoon and onward, I overindulged, gaining weight back and then some. Goals and reasons for losing weight were unrealistic.

An old coworker's situation comes to mind when thinking about people's ridiculous short term goals. This person strongly desired to lose weight for a wedding she was attending. The affair was fancy, a gala in fact. She had a dress custom made for her. It was a "mermaid dress." It was very hip hugging and very narrow below the waist. Think Morticia Addams from *The Addams Family* and you will get a better understanding about the famous mermaid dress. It is tough to walk while wearing this dress, and even more difficult to sit with it on. There was "Linda," a short, stocky woman, dying to fit into a dress that is truly made for tall, thin women.

At lunch, Linda would divulge her diet plans to our jolly group. After all, she had to fit into that dress for the wedding…in three weeks! Of course this is an unreasonable period of time to lose significant amounts of weight. The lot of us highly doubted that her goals would ever be reached in such a short period of time.

Some of Linda's meals consisted of an apple and some water.

Other times she would get a chicken salad sandwich from the cafeteria and would eat half of it. This would seem logical, and of course healthy, but it wasn't if you knew about our cafeteria's chicken salad sandwich. First of all, the unhealthy white bread was slathered with a more than generous amount of mayonnaise. That alone is extremely fattening. The chicken salad itself was a concoction of ingredients, with mayonnaise as the most abundant. This mayonnaise did not just coat the chicken. It looked like the chicken was suspended in a sea of white goo. Whether it was a half a sandwich or whole, it was very high in calories and fat.

"I'm going to eat half a sandwich now, and then have the other half for dinner," Linda announced. "I will lose the weight and look stunning in time for the wedding."

"Gee, I hope you don't outshine the bride," my friend Archino said sarcastically. As an aside, Archino was a good friend of mine. I admired him for his generosity, but for his candor. He told it like it is, holding nothing back. Archino was an elderly man who had the right balance of feistiness and gentleness. (He unfortunately passed away two years later from a long illness. I do miss him.)

The next day, Linda had coffee with us, prattling on about the wonderful dinner she had at her daughter's house.

"Hey, what about that half a sandwich you were going to eat for dinner?" inquired Archino.

"Oh, I ate that too," confessed Linda.

"You mean to tell me that you ate that sandwich and ate at your daughter's house?" accosted Archino. "That's your diet? Well then honey, they are going to have to wrap two dresses around you at the rate you are going."

My jaw dropped and the others snickered. Linda looked ashamed. I quickly changed the subject to diffuse any sad feelings. What did happen was that the dress did not fit well. Linda did not succeed in losing the "required" weight to fit into that dress. Pictures revealed that Linda looked like a stuffed sausage. She confessed to me, when Archino was not around, that she had to stand against a wall during the sit down dinner. She was not able to sit in the dress! She knew if she would try, it would surely rip. How embarrassing!

Linda never lost the weight, then or in the future. Her goals were unrealistic and too short term. She was always trying to lose weight for an event that was coming up in the near future. Her goal was never to lose weight for life. Short term goals fail, making people think that they can never lose weight, and quit as a result. They fail to realize that short term goals are not pursued the right way and the goals themselves are nearly impossible to reach.

The goal should not be to lose weight for a particular event, but for a particular life, your life. Losing weight and adopting a healthier lifestyle should be forever.

Now that we know to avoid quick short term goals, we can focus on losing weight at a decent pace without rushing. Unfortunately certain commercials impact us, making us feel abnormal if the pounds do not just quickly melt away. These dreaded commercials could be so intimidating. "Joe Weightlossguy" lost thirty pounds in a month! "Penny Poundsdrop" lost ten pounds in her first week! When we try to duplicate that kind of rapid weight loss, most of us become really disappointed; we do not drop the weight as quickly as those bragging in commercials. Sometimes we want to pounds to drop quickly, as previously mentioned for short term goals. These goals, as we now know, are ridiculous and should be avoided. Goals should be long term and sustainable. Some of us however, want to have the same success as those who are part of the advertising package. We sometimes measure ourselves against them. If we do not have success equivalent to them, we are failures. Many will give up as a result and go back to old, horrible eating habits.

One of the keys to my weight loss/toning success is that I took the weight off slowly and did not have time constraints. The purpose of losing weight was not for an event or short term thing. This was to be a lifestyle change! I do remember losing five pounds my first week, and about three pounds the second week. After that, the weight loss fluctuated. Sometimes I lost a pound in one week, sometimes a half a pound. Sometimes I lost a quarter of a pound. Sometimes no weight was lost. Sometimes I gained a half of a pound or pound for whatever reason. (Of course with knee surgeries and vacations, I gained more, but I am really focusing on the average week.) Slowly losing the pounds helped me creep up more and more in success.

Many people have asked me how I lost over 100 pounds and did not have loose skin as a result. The answer is that I took the weight off slowly, so my body had "time" to adjust. Little by little I lost the weight, which allowed my body to slowly get in shape. I am sure if I went on a ridiculous diet that led to rapid, temporary weight loss, I would have had saggy skin as a result.

It is best to look at the little picture, taking portions of a pound at a time. If someone told me at the beginning of my weight loss journey that I would have to lose over 100 pounds to be a decent weight, I would have quit right then and there. The number 100 is a massive one, and I would have quit on the spot, claiming it is too difficult. I would think it would take me forever. I would think of my past attempts to lose less than that. I failed at lower weight loss goals, so it would be easy for me to believe that there would be no way to reach this massive goal. Therefore, look at the smaller picture and lose gradually.

CHAPTER 11

Set Goals, Make Commitments

Now that we have short term goals kicked to the curb, it is time to make long term goals that will be achieved and will yield results that last a lifetime! There are many goals we must set to further our progress. If goals and dedication to these goals are not met, there is no guidance and we aimlessly go through the motions, getting little to no results. The week flies by and we find ourselves not doing a bit of what we pledged to do. It is best to start small, making attainable goals. Here are/were some of mine to give you ideas:

- I need to exercise at least three days a week for thirty minutes or more per day. (Proudly, I must say that I increased my workouts to five days a week, an hour minimum. If I began with the five days a week goal, an hour a day, I would have surely failed. Therefore, the goals have to be small at first!)

- I want to tone my abdomen, so I will aim for 50 crunches a day for three days a week. (Now I do 500 crunches a day for four days a week).

- I will try to eat fewer calories than the day before. (This goal pertains to those counting calories and you are in a higher caloric intake range. Consult with a doctor first.)

- I will reduce the number of times I dine out from three times a week to once a week. (This was a tough goal since I was eating take - out food all weekend long while working.)

- I will split my desserts with my friend/spouse/child or at least take half of it home.

- I will increase my time on the treadmill/elliptical machine from 15 minutes to 17 minutes. (Now I am on the treadmill/ elliptical machine for 45 minutes.)

- I will increase the resistance on the _(insert machine name here)_ from _(insert original resistance setting here)_ to _(insert new original resistance setting here)._ Make sure the increase is only by one increment.

- My inner thighs/arms/other areas need(s) toning. I will research what exercises are best for the target area(s). (Hint: For tips, use the internet, books, a personal trainer, or a doctor.)

- I need to have fruit as one of my desserts each day. It could be a lunch or dinner dessert. I cannot have cookies or other processed foods for both lunch and dinner desserts.

Setting goals for eating habits, problem areas, and exercising will help you see results. Just aimlessly walking around the block or on a treadmill may produce some results at first, but will not be long lasting. We have to be mindful of what we are doing and improve what we are doing to see results. After a time, our body gets used to it. Our fifteen minutes of exercise, for example, will no longer contribute to weight loss. An increase in time will, and that would work best if the increase was gradual. Noting our problems and finding solutions will put us on the path to success.

CHAPTER 12

Stop the Shoveling and Stuffing

Now that goals are set and commitments are made, we can now turn our attention to the food in our hands. One of the biggest problems we face with our eating habits is shoveling food in our mouths at a fast pace. Some of us know that it takes time for the message of fullness to be sent to the brain. In the meantime, more food is shoved into our systems, more than we obviously need to feel full. For some, eating quickly makes them feel that they really did not eat much. After all, look how quickly the meal was consumed. Each feels deprived and grabs seconds or some kind of snack food right after eating a meal. A great many of us end up overstuffed, bloated, and sluggish. Excuses for this terrible habit are justified by lack of time. We all have busy lifestyles. Our jobs, families, chores, and errands occupy a huge chunk of our time. People tend to "wolf down" their food so they can go on to the next task or destination.

What is the solution? Is it to keep doing this? After all, the excuse is that we are busy, so we have to eat quickly. The answer is to drop the excuse! Eating quickly is one of the reasons for weight gain, so there has to be modifications in our lifestyle. Eating at a slower pace will not consume a tremendous amount of time. Taking even three to five minutes more to eat a meal is doable for most of us; it is not as bad as you think.

My helpful tools are a shrimp fork and a baby spoon/teaspoon. Not only does it disallow me from piling heaping amounts of food on the utensils, but it allows me to savor my food more. Hey, if I am putting a certain amount of calories and fat into my system, I should at least be able to enjoy every morsel! Most restaurants have big utensils as the standard, especially the spoons. They are so large, that they almost seem to be mini shovels. It is too tempting to load it up with lots of food and shovel it into my mouth. Therefore, at restaurants, I request the smallest spoons and forks they have. Sometimes restaurants have small tea spoons, which work quite nicely. Some long handled iced tea spoons have smaller "bowls" to scoop food than standard spoons that are given. Most restaurants can accommodate the smaller utensil request, especially seafood eateries. Though rare, if the request cannot be fulfilled, I simply make sure to eat slow and not load my utensils with food. I make sure my utensil is not fully loaded with food, but only contains a small portion. This involves a great deal of concentration. When dining out with family and friends, it is easy to pile food on and in without truly noticing what is being eaten. So try to simultaneously focus on friends, family, and food quantities at the end of your fork or spoon.

To broaden your variety of utensils, use chopsticks for those special meals. Of course this recommendation is not for everyone. Some get frustrated while eating with them, which of course spoils the dining experience. For others, utilizing chopsticks is a dining adventure! However, some foods are not meant to be eaten with chopsticks. Soups are first to come to mind but I am sure you can think of other things. For those who are not pros in eating with chopsticks, try it out. It may slow eating down and even make it an adventurous experience. For those who get frustrated easily, calmly put the chopsticks away or donate them to a grateful recipient!

To make the meal last longer, cut the food into smaller pieces as you eat. As an example, I cut each shrimp or scallop into three pieces that I eat separately. Most people pop an entire shrimp or scallop into their mouths. The food needs to be smaller, last longer, and needs to be eaten slower!

"Speaking" of eating slower, another way to eat slowly is to eat with your non dominant hand. Most of us are not ambidextrous, so it takes us longer to do a task when using our non dominant or non writing hand. Eating is one of those tasks. Try it! You will see that it takes longer to eat. It is another great way to slow eating down!

Another way to make my meal last is to eat one sandwich half at a time. For instance, I will not bite into two pieces of bread of my peanut butter and strawberry sandwich. I still spread the same amount, but on two separate pieces of bread. Eating one piece at a time tricks me into being more satisfied. Doing this allows me to eat a lot slower, feeling full faster. It also tricks me into believing that I ate much more.

A final strategy is use a small fork and a knife for foods that are normally eaten with our hands. This includes pizza, burgers, tacos, wraps/sandwiches, fajitas, cannolis, and the like. I eat a burger with my shrimp fork and knife. It lasts longer and I get to savor it. It is better than taking huge bites. I enjoy eating fajitas with a shrimp fork and knife. I can actually taste the chicken or steak better and get more of a full flavor. I can also taste the ingredients I put into it more such as sour cream and/or cheese in small amounts. I really do savor my meals more by eating this way; the tastes are more detected because I am taking the time to taste instead of being a glutton. I end up eating less in the long run, getting fuller faster. Remember, the quicker you eat, the more food you will stuff yourself with. It is better to eat with small utensils than taking massive bites of food. If utensils are not readily available, try to be conscious of the amount of food taken in. Make sure bites are small.

Another bad habit that goes hand in hand with the shoveling is stuffing. We all have done this. For instance, we see a bowl or bag of popcorn or pretzels. We reach in and grab massive amounts to stuff our faces with these crunchy treats. There are two problems with this. The first is that we are stuffing ourselves quickly before signals can get to our brains to let us know we are full. The second is that we do not feel satisfied with a small amount.

I encountered this problem while trying to lose weight. I would measure two cups of popcorn. Before I knew it, my two cups were gone super fast.

"That's it?" I would question myself. I didn't feel satisfied and wanted to reach for more.

Being a forward thinker and problem solver, I came up with a way to enjoy the amount that was measured out. I ate one kernel of popcorn at a time and savored each one. As mentioned previously, chopsticks are a great tool. It slows down the eating and the treat can be enjoyed more for its great taste. Try this or simply eat one piece at a time, savoring every morsel. Don't use an excuse about not being able to do so. Don't say it is impossible for you, that you just have to pop more food in your mouth. Try it, think about the food you are eating, and savor it. There is white/dark chocolate covered popcorn that I budget in my diet from time to time. I measured one and a half cups of it. Yes, I do treat myself! I don't always eat healthy all the time because I am human like everyone else! I like a treat just like the next person. What I can say is that I eat healthy MOST of the time! Treating myself once in awhile helps me to stick to healthy eating. Therefore, I splurge for the chocolate covered popcorn from time to time. I eat one kernel at a time of this magnificent popcorn, savoring that amazing chocolate. I allow it to melt in my mouth. It is more satisfying than gobbling it down quickly and wondering where it all went soon after.

If I am eating ice cream, whether in my home or at an ice cream parlor, I always make sure to eat it with a small spoon. If I am at an ice cream parlor, I ask for a sample spoon. Some places have small spoons that they use to give samples to customers who want to try a flavor before buying. These small spoons are most ideal to eat ice cream with. I stick to ice cream in a cup and never eat ice cream in a cone. The ice cream is fattening enough and has enough calories. I do not need extra calories and fat that an ice cream cone brings. Additionally, ice cream in a cone has to be consumed quicker before it drips and becomes messy. Eating ice cream in a cup gives more control and fewer calories, sans the cone. We can then eat ice cream at a slower pace, using a small spoon.

Additionally, make sure you eat without distractions. Watching television, talking, reading, and writing are some activities that distract. You do not realize what you are eating or how much. Concentrate on the food in hand!

CHAPTER 13

Beverages and Coffee Chemistry

Most of us who want to lose weight focus on what we eat. We also must be mindful of what we drink. Beverages can add a great deal of calories and fat to a diet. Some drinks add a lot of sugar and unnecessary chemicals as well. Many alcoholic beverages add a great deal of calories and chemicals to our diets. Some sodas add a lot of sugar and chemicals. We could end up drinking lots of chemical concoctions. Some people drink these in massive quantities on a daily basis. Eliminating or greatly reducing the consumption of these kinds of drinks alone can truly jumpstart weight loss.

My beverage of choice is water. I realize that some people cannot drink water alone, and need some flavor. As always, I have an alternative plan. Put a lemon or orange slice in the water. It is so fancy to do so, as ritzy restaurants often serve water this way. For more flavor, squeeze some of the lemon or orange juice into the water. Another option is to take strawberries and blend it into the water. The number of strawberries to add depends on the preferred intensity of the flavor. I usually like ice water with a tinge of strawberry flavor, so I would blend one strawberry into an eight ounce glass of water.

Some people do not get enough fruit into their diets. For these people, I recommend one cup of fruit juice, but diluted. Mix one cup of juice with a half a cup of water. Have one of these drinks per day, as many have too much juice on a daily basis.

If you want to be adventurous, try drinking carrot juice. Many grimace at the mention of this drink, but never tried it. It is very satisfying, and has a tinge of sweetness. The right brand has the right flavor. I recommend the refrigerated carrot juice. Try not to buy brands, both carrot juice and carrot juice blends, that are sitting on the shelf at room temperature. Fresher is better! For those with juicers, dust them off and get to juicing!

Various articles and books point out that drinking at least six 8oz glasses of water daily is beneficial to weigh loss/maintenance. Do try for at least six glasses. Work it into the day. Besides, drinking more water reduces hunger, and you will be less out to binge.

Try to eliminate the chemical concoctions and go for healthier alternatives. Not only are they better for weight loss, they are better for your health.

Now we can tackle the coffee chemistry. I know there are a lot of people out there who just have to have coffee every morning. Why do you think Starbucks and Dunkin Donuts are faring well? Yours truly is a coffee fanatic. Coffee or even tea alone does not cause people to gain weight. The problem is that sugar and cream could really pack on the calories and fat. Also, specialty coffees, especially the ones topped with whipped cream, are fattening. There are some modifications you can make and still enjoy that cup of coffee or tea without making drastic changes to the amazing taste.

The key is to order a basic coffee or tea that is "natural" and does not have the consistency of a milkshake! Let us first start with the sugar/sweetener portion. If you want to stick to natural sugar, try your coffee or tea with less and less sugar each time. Start with a measured amount, and reduce by small increments each time. Eventually, you will get used to using less sugar. Adding a flavored coffee creamer like hazelnut or French vanilla could compensate for that loss of sweetness. Just the right balance could get you just the right enjoyment with less sugar. Honey is also an amazing sugar substitute, even in coffee. If using a sugar substitute, choose the "healthiest" one. At the time of this publishing, there are mixed reviews of sugar substitutes. Some have been known to cause cancer (i.e. saccharine), and others have findings that are mixed or inconclusive. Regardless, sugar substitutes should not be heavily depended on. I personally use regular sugar (sparingly) because I try to take a more natural route when I can.

Now let us examine the milk portion. If you drink your coffee or tea "black" or without milk, then you do not have to worry about this portion. However, if you like your beverage creamy like I do, then you need to find options which have fewer fat and calories. Most coffee houses have three types of milk: half and half, whole milk, and one or two percent milk. Why not mix all three? Mixing this would reduce calories and fat compared to straight half and half. I try to put more one percent milk into the coffee first, adding more of the milk that has the fewest calories and grams of fat. I then follow it by the whole milk. By the time I get to the half and half, there is not as much room for it in my coffee. Therefore, there is little space for the most fattening milk. After all is added, the coffee tastes just as good and is satisfying. Mentally, you will be satisfied because the fattening creamer is in the coffee.

So do a little coffee or tea chemistry. Sometimes it takes a few "experiments" to get it to taste right, but the right combination will be second nature once identified. Be a chemist - try healthier combinations that will not contribute to adding on the pounds!

CHAPTER 14

Party of Fat in and out of Your Home

So many parties, so much to do! Some of us love to attend certain parties, some do not. Just seeing negative people who annoy us in one way or another is enough for some of us to pig out to "kill the pain." Some of us reach for alcohol, and some of us reach for the food. And hey, there is so much to indulge on! Stress or no stress, there are too many excuses to eat, especially if there is a lot of tempting food. If a party is held in your own home, food is easier to control. Realistically, parties are mostly outside of our homes. They are at relatives' homes, friends' homes, workplaces, restaurants, and catering halls. Sometimes parties are sporadic; sometimes they come in clusters, especially during November and December. Regardless of the type of party, regardless of the location, regardless of the party frequencies, I know how to handle them. I want you to learn to handle yourself too!

I want to first "shoot down" a worthless piece of advice I have read over and over again regarding parties in and out of the home. Even talk shows offer the same piece of advice. The "helpful" tip is to have a small meal before the party commences. No, no, no, no, no! Never eat a small meal before a party! The logic behind this advice is that eating before a party will allow the person to feel full and not feel the urge to pig out at a party. Are we talking fantasy here? I don't know about you, but I tried this and still managed to stuff myself with the tempting foods I saw. I made room for the mini hot dogs, mini pizzas, mini eggrolls, quiches, pasta dishes, chicken parmesan, cheddar mashed potatoes, prime rib, rice, éclairs, chocolate mousse, cheesecake, and even a nice cappuccino. I always managed to find foods that I just had to sample. My stomach gladly made room for them all, regardless of the small meal from before. Therefore, I took in calories from my small meal and my party meal - or should I say party meals?

I had to modify the way I approached parties. If I am hosting, I make them commence in the early afternoon, around 2 or 2:30 pm. This would be my "linner" time, a combination of lunch and dinner. Therefore my calories would account for lunch and dinner. There is an added benefit in having this "linner," which is that you only end up serving one meal. When I used to serve lunch, people would stay late and I would have to continue serving food for dinner. It was an all day serving affair. This mid afternoon time is ideal for just serving one meal, making less work for all involved.

I must be clear and say that I am not one to promote skipping meals. Everyone should have balanced breakfasts, lunches, and dinners. For those with medical issues, snacks are often necessary in between meals, and those should check with their doctor before following this advice (or any eating advice). I am not leading you into dangerous/unhealthy waters. I am trying to get you through a party. Skipping meals should not be a regular part of a typical day.

I begin my party with appetizers about fifteen minutes after the first guest arrives. I offer them beverages while I put the appetizers on the designated plates. This gives people a chance to arrive and mingle. My appetizers are not as greasy or unhealthy. I make my own mini pizzas. I will either make my own pizza dough or use the refrigerated kind. I shape small, round pizzas, baking the crusts first, adding the sauce and shredded cheese, and baking them until the cheese is well melted. I make a special mini pizza for me, using less dough and less cheese. Vegetables and dip are also on hand, but the dip is low fat. I include low to no fat dips, including hummus and salsa. Since non-starchy vegetables are unlimited in my healthy eating plan, I can pig out on vegetables and low fat/no fat dips.

If I am having a small party for just my husband, son, and myself, I will serve something light for myself at noon and serve a small sandwich for the boys. These items will tide us over for our 2 or 2:30 meal. The lighter fare for me could include a salad with a few garbanzo beans in it for fiber and for the contribution to my fullness.

When I host a party, I make very sure I keep busy. This includes chatting, serving, and cleaning. Keeping busy eliminates time to delve into the fattening foods I do have out. Running around to cook, serve, clean, and entertain overall is also great exercise. There is always a good food choice for me. Entrees are healthy. Meats and poultry are not in creamy/fatty sauces. Vegetables are always on hand. At the end of this chapter, I will list some healthy choices.

Desserts have to be good. I do serve fattening desserts. Fruit and gelatin desserts will not cut it for my guests. I do serve cheesecake, chocolate cake, apple crisp, and homemade ice cream. If possible, have a separate portion already dished out. I take a half a slice of cheesecake and keep it aside for me. Guests are able to take as much or as little as they want. I need to portion my dessert out ahead of time. I know if I serve myself along with everyone else, I will not be honest with myself. If they take a huge slab of cake, then I want a mega huge piece too. Another option would be to have a healthier dessert on hand. See recipe sections to get a few ideas for healthier dessert options. Make extra for those who may be interested in a better option or for those who simply want to try it.

Some of you may be pondering the question as to why I am separating out portions and leaving everyone else eat higher calories, higher fat foods. Let us face it, not everyone eats like us. If I fed my guests what I normally eat, they would be really disappointed. Some are not watching their weight - sometimes it shows on them and sometimes it doesn't. Others do not have to worry about their portions - they eat a lot and do not gain thanks to their super miraculous metabolism. Some watch what they eat, but want to splurge once in awhile when at a party. I cannot be a killjoy. Most of the foods are healthy and people are free to eat as much or as little as they want. I cannot police my friends and outside the house family. Carrot sticks and celery just won't cut it and those items would be a sure way to receive many declines to future parties. If you do have guests that are health conscious, by all means, make all portions like yours. Make only healthy food. If there is a mix of people, both health conscious and not, set aside lower fat entrees. For instance, make stuffed shells the "regular way" and some with less ricotta and mozzarella cheese. Tell all guests which is which and let them decide what they want to eat. When it comes down to it, meal choices depend on the party attendees.

If the party is not at your home, do not despair. A mid afternoon party would be best, because like the house party, lunch and dinner can be combined. If the party is later in the evening, have a lighter than usual breakfast and lunch. On party days, I usually have fruit for breakfast. For lunch I eat a piece of wheat toast with a level tablespoon of peanut butter and cut up strawberries. No dessert for lunch - there will be plenty of food for the evening party.

If it is the type of party where appetizers are served, limit yourself to two. This does not mean a full plate of quiche and mini hot dogs. Those are two KINDS of appetizers, not two individual appetizers. Appetizer quantities are individual portions that can be pierced with a toothpick and are "bite - sized." For instance, I will have a mini pizza (three inch diameter pizza) and mini spinach pie triangle (Spanokopita). Then I am done with appetizers. I give myself a break until I have the main course. At least I got a taste of some of the "naughty," greasy items. Having two small appetizers is far better than having ten, believe me! More is not always better. Even if a better appetizer comes along, stay away from it! After two appetizers, you already had your fill. Not keeping track of appetizers can really be bad for you. Settling for two appetizers takes away the guesswork for how many appetizers you actually ate. The old me would chat and grab every appetizer that was presented by a server. I just had to try everything. It got to a point where I couldn't even remember eating so much. One time I was chatting with people at a fancy party, while servers walked around with trays of appetizers. Each item came with a toothpick. When it was time to sit down to dinner, I had ten toothpicks in my hand! That meant ten appetizers that I stuffed my face with, not knowing that I indeed had that many. Thus, appetizers add up quickly, in your face and on your waist!

Another problem most of us have is resisting the snacks in bowls. This includes pretzels, chips, nuts, and the like. The dips that often accompany them can also be fattening, high caloric concoctions. I try to gross myself out so I will not be tempted to eat these kinds of foods. One way I avoid them is to really think about the sanitary part about them. Have you noticed that people who use the rest room oftentimes do not wash their hands? Do you realize that people who arrive just touched their dirty car keys, doors and knobs, and other contaminated things? Then they reach for these bowls of goodies. Most bowls of treats do not have tongs or serving spoons. People are allowed to dip their dirty, grubby hands into it. I one time saw a guest cough into his hands, and then reach for some pretzels with the hand he coughed into. Who needs food coated with germs? I also see the double dipper person, the one who takes a chip, dips it in a dip, takes a bite, and then dips it back into the dip again with his germs and all. Looking at the reality, do you really want these bowls of bacteria? Think about the gross parts about it and I am sure you will be able to stay away from them much easier! See the chapter, *Can You Gross Yourself Out While You are Out?* for more "gross" ideas.

Most parties are self serve. If you are moving through the "buffet line," fill half your plate with a salad and/or vegetables. Do not use a separate plate for the salad. The entire meal, aside from dessert, should fit on one plate. Watch the dressing - a spoonful (not ladle size) will do. One quarter of your plate could be a pasta dish, and the other quarter would be meat/chicken/tofu. Make sure you do not pile up the plate. The food from the plate's side view should not look like a mountain.

One dessert or two mini desserts will be perfect. One slice of cake would be great, but not cake and those cream puffs…haven't had one of them in a long time. Oh, and there's that warm apple crisp, and I have to have a dollop of ice cream to go with that…

If cake with icing is a dessert, especially the kind served at birthday parties, lop off the icing! Sometimes the icing has more calories and fat than the cake part! These cakes are usually two or three layers, so there will be enough icing to taste between the other layers. You certainly do not need icing on top and you will experience the same flavor. There is plenty of icing throughout! Just enjoy the cake and ditch the icing! Taking off the top layer of icing is very beneficial because fewer calories and fat are consumed. Taking it off will make the cake less sweet, which is a good thing; very sweet icing can be overpowering, making the dessert less enjoyable. Sometimes the cake is so rich with thick layers of icing, that I only eat the cake part in between the layers. Therefore, I will avoid the icing altogether. Finally, removing the icing would allow you to remove the most contaminated part of the cake. Most people blow out candles on a birthday cake. Therefore, they are blowing on the cake. When I was a scientist years ago, we did an experiment where we blew in a Petri dish. Long story short, we were able to grow colonies and colonies of bacteria, just from what we blew in this dish. In short, when people blow on a cake, they are depositing their germs. Some families relight the candles and have the youngest children blow out the candles. Then there is a potpourri of germs on the cake. The trick candles that do not blow out easily make the person try to blow harder and more often. Now there are more germs than average on the cake. To me, it is a "spit cake." Taking off the icing, the protective coating, is definitely a good thing. (By the way, we light separate candles, and do not place them on the cake. That ensures a "spit free" cake!) Therefore, icing can be your friend, but not for eating! That could have a bad effect on your waist. Look at it as a protective coating or protective layer for the cake. Remove and enjoy the cake part, ingesting no spit whatsoever and fewer germs, calories, and fat!

The aforementioned tips are for those parties that have a few healthy entrees. Unfortunately there are those who serve nothing but unhealthy foods. I have seen "grease fests" of foods that are nothing but bad news for my weight! These homes are well known to me now, so there is no surprise as to what to expect. In that case, I will lightly "graze" to be polite. I will have a small amount of food. Later on, I will eat a healthier meal that I packed in an insulated lunch bag in the car. If the party is not far from home, I will simply wait; there is more of a meal choice in my own kitchen!

Another option is to bring a healthy dish. A vegetable tray is something that is easy to graze from. A healthy pasta dish can be easy to make (e.g. baked ziti sans lots of cheese). You know what is in it and know it is okay to have. Bringing a healthy dessert will also be beneficial. Good dessert choices include fruit salad, brownies, with little/no icing, fruit kebabs, or chocolate pudding made with skim milk. Sometimes I will bring a frozen gourmet cheesecake; I know the calories and fat per slice. Depending on the amount of calories and fat, I will either have a half or full slice. At least I do not have to second guess a dessert.

You may appear nice enough to bring food, but in reality, you are also helping yourself. You need not second guess the fat and calorie content of someone else's food. You know exactly what is in each dish you bring.

Be sure to try recipes from the Ravishing Recipes chapter. With small changes, you can indeed handle the party of fat! Read on to see how your party can be set up healthy!

Salad

Have lots of it - half a plate, remember? Include a variety of greens and other salad accompaniments. Make sure you have on hand most of the following:

Lettuce	tomatoes	garbanzo beans
cucumbers	green olives	(a.k.a. chick peas)
dried cherries	green/red peppers	
onions	black olives	

Have fattening dressings on hand for those who want to indulge. My favorite low - cal dressings that taste fattening are the following:

- Trader Joe's Champagne Pear Vinaigrette - at a mere 45 calories and 2.5 grams of fat for a two tablespoon serving, this dressing is both healthy and flavorful.
- Most Japanese ginger dressings. Most are low in calories and fat. Check them out!
- Most raspberry/strawberry vinaigrette dressings. Again, check labels.

My own quick dressing version:

- 1 cup cut strawberries
- 1 tsp sugar
- 2 tsp raspberry vinegar or red wine vinegar. Combine ingredients. Use a potato masher to blend. Dressing should be on the chunky side.

Vegetable Sides

Make cooked side vegetables with no seasonings. Have salt, pepper, butter, and margarine close by to have guests season to their liking. Invite them to the seasonings. People can be picky anyway. Some do not like a lot of salt on vegetables, some do. Some enjoy lots of butter or margarine, some do not. Giving a choice allows people to season to their liking.

Dessert

There are many options for dessert. See the chapter on bulking up dessert. It is easy to serve ice cream with fruit mixed in. See the Recipe Renovation and Ravishing Recipes chapters also; the former gives tips on how to reduce calories and fat of beloved recipes by making simple modifications.

CHAPTER 15

Let Your Clothes and Scale Be Your Leash

I do not mean anything bad by comparing myself or anyone else to a dog. However, the way I look at clothes makes the image complete for me. Fitted clothes, that is, clothes without elastic or much give, is like a leash for me. If I eat too much very frequently, my clothes pull on me. They pull me back, and make me go where I should, just as a leash does for a dog. The tightness of the clothes constricts and reminds me to get back on track and eat right. This holds me back so I do not get carried away, especially at parties or restaurants.

Another option that can be used in place of or in addition to the clothes is the belt itself. The belt is helpful if it is a little tight when dining out. The pull the belt has around the waist signals the individual that enough is enough. It is time to stop eating. It is a nifty tool that I have had to use from time to time. This can help with longer goals as well, to make sure our eating isn't out of control for long. Note the notch that the belt is usually fastened on. If it gets to a point in which the belt can no longer be comfortably fastened on that notch, it is time to reexamine current eating and exercising practices. It is clear that there is weight gain and changes need to be made. If we are not mindful of these things, not having any restrictions as indications, we will gain and notice when the difference is indeed too significant.

I must caution the overachievers NOT to tighten the belt to a ridiculous degree. Please do not make your belts too tight. The belt should be snug, but not insanely constricting. You should be able to move and breathe freely! If the belt is simply snug, you can still tell the difference and feel the tightness if you consume too much food.

Try to wear fitted clothes as opposed to clothes that have a lot of give. This includes elastic waist jeans, pants, skirts, and shorts. It is difficult to tell if weight is gained if clothes have a lot of that flexibility. The old person I used to be wore pants with elastic. At one point I gained thirty pounds and did not even know it. It may seem kind of obvious to recognize such a weight gain, but not for me. My clothes were baggy and stretchy. Nothing was tight, and the baggy clothes did not show my weight gain. I never dared looked at myself in a mirror, either naked or partially clothed. My reflection disgusted me so much, so I never discovered the extra pounds until much later. The baggy shirts and elastic pants did not help me see the major weight gain. Those types of clothes simply stretch to accommodate growing size. If I wore tighter clothes, I would have noticed the difference, and perhaps would have started getting back on track sooner.

My current pants/jeans size ranges from a 4 to a 6, depending on the style. This is honestly a good size for me due to my body structure. I make sure that I stay in this range, and do not easily accommodate myself by wearing a larger size. If the jeans are a little snug, I know to get back on track; it is a little reminder to get back to healthy eating.

Be sure to wear fitted clothes regularly. Do not make it a "sometime" ritual. It is upsetting and more defeating to try on a pair of jeans, only to find that the button does not even fasten around the waist. This results from occasionally wearing fitted clothes. Do not get to that point. Fitted clothes helps keep us in check. If we get carried away with food, these clothes let us know, pushing us towards getting back on track and "getting it right."

The scale can also act as a "leash." It indicates whether or not we are losing/gaining/maintaining. I would utilize this tool wisely. Some obsess over the scale if there is a 0.2 pound gain. We should not get upset over minute changes. It should not be a tool of torture! I weigh myself each morning but use the numbers on the scale as a light guide. Weight fluctuates, so I will not get upset if I am up a pound. Now that I am at goal weight, I am sure to keep my weight to a five pound range. When I was still losing weight, I understood that there can be days of weight gain, but knew it was a "red flag" when the weight gain was significant. If that occurred, I knew the reason or reasons most of the time. For instance, the party or the holiday the day before was the contributing factor. If you are obsessed with the scale, choose a day and just weigh yourself once a week on that day. The scale can be your "leash" because the numbers could help you hold back on unhealthy eating. It can also motivate to exercise more or make better choices overall.

The clothes and scale are great tools to help keep you in check and keep you on the right track!

CHAPTER 16

Variety of Exercise is the Spice of Life

$\mathcal{E}$xercise is a major factor in my life. If I didn't do it, I would not get the results I currently have. Though everyone is different, I would have to say that we would all be bored if we did the same exercise on a daily basis. I am one of these people. Boring exercises can lead to quitting, which will yield failure to get and remain on the healthy track. I have many suggestions about how to get spice out of your exercise. Some may be doable for some and not for others. And of course always check with your doctor before beginning any exercise program. Here are some suggestions. Just pick and choose what would work best for you, your body, and of course, your budget.

Try a gym to get out and work out! Not all gyms are expensive. Some even have a free week or even a trial month. I strongly recommend trying out a gym before making a solid commitment. Do not be shy to call several gyms and get pricing. Over the years, I delved into gyms. This was a huge mistake. Some work-out establishments have a snobby "atmosphere." One place I tried out had a very friendly worker who showed me around and signed me up. She acted like she was my best friend. After signing up, I walked by the desk two days later, and said hello to her. She looked at me with disgust and turned her head. I guess I was good enough to speak to when I joined the club, but after that, being friendly to me was not an option. One gym did not like my overweight mother sitting by the window in the waiting room. I guess it wasn't good for their image if people walked by the window and saw an overweight person sitting there. They made her wait in the child care room. I returned from my workout to find she was gone. I was told she wasn't allowed to WAIT in the WAITING room! They had her sit on a folding chair in the middle of the room while little kids played around her. My mom was a good sport, but the sight was demeaning and made me cry. It was belittling to the both of us, and I never returned. I lost a great deal of money on that one. Another gym would not allow me to use the weight lifting equipment because staff members said I should only take classes to get the fat off first, then tone. Employees who saw me use the equipment told me that I was too overweight to tone and I should lose weight first before using the machines. I couldn't believe they actually stopped me from using the machines. I paid for a full membership, not a class only membership. I should have been free to use what I wished.

I worked out at a gym that was great for a period of time and I loved it! I knew it was for me when there was no pressure or gimmicks when I came to visit. I was able to go to the gym all awful looking, and no one judged me. Because I was there quite a bit, I knew a lot of the "regulars." We had become a kind of family, which was beautiful to me. So many had cheered me on during my weight loss journey, from the trainers to the members. There was always someone to chat with, whether on a cardio machine or in the locker room. I also had some variety in machines and overall things to do. I was able to use the elliptical machine or treadmill. I could then go bench press or get the mat to do sit ups. I could use the exercise ball for crunches or other types of exercise. I could take a boot camp class or Pilates class. Because of the two cracks in my right kneecap, I am unable to kneel. This does not stop me from taking a class. I made modifications and did something different from the rest. The instructors knew my story and just let me do what I can do. I could ride a stationary bike or even take a spin class. There were also swimming and even aerobic swim classes that were free to members. Listening to music during my workouts really got me to move much more!

Taking exercise classes at the gym or elsewhere is a great way to get variety. Some classes are held in dance studios and are open to the public. I have even seen Zumba classes held in the evenings at libraries! There are also places that are exclusive to exercise classes like exercise class studios. It is a good way to switch things up, try something fresh, and exercise different parts of the body. A trick I use once I am comfortable in the class is to exercise in the front row. This makes me try a little harder instead of being languid in the back. Exercising towards the front gives me more energy and I tend to try harder. It is similar to the effect of sitting at the front of the classroom. The attention span is higher and students tend to try harder.

Some people may need a variety when it comes to working out. If you exercise in your home, switch rooms. Some may even want to switch gyms once the membership is expired. Gyms are so very different. Exercising at a new gym may bring variety, new exercise equipment/exercise classes that were not at the old gym. The new atmosphere alone can be pleasing and motivating. Some people do not like variety and that is okay. It is worth trying in order to keep motivation up and boredom to a nonexistent level.

I really did enjoy working out at one gym, but after many years, I felt like a hamster running around in a wheel. It was the same boring routine. I could not get variety any longer due to the crowded gym. I was limited to thirty minutes on cardio machines due to the overwhelming demand. I ended up doing the same things, having the same routine. Though I loved that gym, I ventured out for a change. I was fortunate enough to find a gym that had more cardio machines, more classes, and no time limits on equipment. There were also nice little amenities that the other gym did not have. Therefore, I got more variety and lots of nice little bonuses. These factors helped me stick to my goal and tone even more.

Depending on your lifestyle, you may want to choose a gym closer to your workplace. Sadly, I had to leave that gym near my home where I had "family" because my work and son's school concentrated me in a totally different county! Transferring to another gym allowed me to travel less and exercise more.

If you are not a fan of venturing out and you have some spare cash, invest in a mini gym that does not take up a lot of space in vital areas of your home. Invest in exercise videos and maybe two pieces of exercise equipment. You can even rent a variety of exercise videos from the library or even view some on the internet. People are always selling exercise equipment because it is taking up space. That is a good way to get equipment at a lower price. Some quit so easily, so the exercise equipment is barely used. So look at flea markets, garage sales, and ads in local papers and bulletin boards. If you rent videos, perhaps rent some of these exercise DVD's/Blue Ray/whatever technology is out….This trial basis can help you see if this is good for you. Exercise equipment is a matter of preference. It all depends on what is fun for you to do. A treadmill would be ideal in case weather does not cooperate for a walk. An elliptical machine would also be great to have, but it depends on preference. Both pieces of equipment range from reasonable to very expensive in price. These two pieces of equipment are mere suggestions; there are a lot of machines out there and it all comes down to choice. If space is an issue, try to find equipment that folds up. Perhaps setting up a gym in the basement would be better.

Though I frequent a gym, there is still a wide array of exercise "equipment" in my home. There are several workout VHS tapes and

DVDs that I use. If I am snowed in, I can easily pop in a video. If I only have a few minutes to workout, these videos are ideal. I can stop them at anytime. I have a few dance games discs that can be utilized on my son's video game system. The system has exercise games and even a Zumba game! They make for nice workouts and do give a lot of variety.

Going for walks is sensational. It too gives variety. I change my course so I do not see the same sights. Even walking in the mall is great. Some malls have an early morning walking club, which is a great way to meet people. The mall is completely quiet, so it is nice to walk around, do window shopping, and enjoy silence. Can you believe that I actually enjoy walking in the mall? When I was at my highest weight, I hated walking. Now I park in far away spots and try to walk as much as I can. Walking in the mall is now fun for me!

Make it a game! One way I do so is with my pedometer. Do invest in one. They are not that expensive. I will always try to beat my record from the previous day. I always want to walk more steps than the day before. Maybe you want to even record your exercise time and try to beat that record. Perhaps you want to do more repetitions in a particular exercise. I did that with crunches. At first, I started with 100. I now do between 500 to 600 crunches a day!

Losing weight made me feel very youthful at heart. This sparked me to do something "crazy," taking a tap class. I used to take an adult tap class at the dance studio that my son attended. We got to dance in the same recital, but not, of course, in the same dances. Tapping is another way to get in my exercise, and it is so much fun. Additionally, I take a Zumba class from time to time. For those who are not familiar with this type of class, Zumba incorporates Latin dance into the workout. It is like a dance aerobics. It is so much fun for me. I am lucky to find classes that are so much fun and so healthy for me too. I am burning calories doing things that I love. You need to find fun things too and go for it!

My husband is not a dancer, but something inside him ventured into doing a Zumba video with me. He was surprised that he was able to do the steps and catch up. As a family, we even do a Zumba class on my son's video game system. My husband now loves it. He really thought he would hate it, but gave it a try. Even if you think you will hate something, give it a shot. Try new things! The better the variety, the less the boredom with exercise!

Now that variety is covered, keep in mind to target certain areas you would like to tone. I have had so many people approach me to inquire about my weight loss journey. In this conversation, most complain that they cannot tone a particular area. Many pinch the area that needs work. People will pinch the front of the gut and say, "See, I have this gut to lose and I can't tone it." I ask them if they do any exercises to target their area. Their answer is always no! What? You are complaining about flab and you do no exercise whatsoever to tone it? How will it go away? By eating right alone? By magic? By a magic fat begone pill?

If you belong to a local gym, tell the trainers about where you want to tone and then ask for some exercise recommendations. The internet is also a valuable source of information for exercise suggestions. Some websites have instructional videos. Some famous exercise gurus have websites that offer toning suggestions. Let's not forget about books that offer advice and illustrations to help get on the right track. If unsure, ask your doctor if a specific exercise is right for you, especially if there is an existing problem.

If you are going to join a gym or already belong to a gym, take advantage of the exercise classes that are offered. I highly recommend these classes. First, it satisfies the variety component that is needed for any exercise regimen. Second, it drives people to do more exercise than if they exercised alone. I personally know that I will not do as many repetitions by myself. When I am in the class, I want to keep up, so I push on. Third, classes often help with toning to some degree. What you must be aware of is that you cannot rely on a class to take care of target areas you want to sculpt. For instance, if you need to tone your stomach, the amount of abdominal exercises done in the class will not help tone it the way you desire. This is especially true if it is a class that works on a little bit of everything, or does five minutes of abdominals at the end of whatever class it is. Sometimes a little more toning is necessary and that must be done on your own. You must personally sculpt the area of interest. And sculpting involves at least three times a week. Working on a target area once a week will not yield noticeable results. For instance, if abdominals are the target area, do them three times a week. A once a week abs class will just not cut it. Therefore, find ways to tone where you want. Remember, it will not be tone by diet alone!

CHAPTER 17

Lose the Weight While You Wait

As you can see, variety in your exercise is one of the keys to success. Keep it interesting, keep it exciting. But did you know you can get variety in exercise while you are waiting for things? The reality is that in this busy, hustle and bustle world, we do a lot of waiting, we wait, wait, and wait some more. We wait a long time in line at the supermarket. People with full carts are ahead of us, or the famous jerks who have fifty items in a ten items or less lane suck up a lot of our time. Let us not forget the pains who have some sort of issue with a price or payment, forcing the cashier to get extra help from another staff member. We wait with our kids at the curb for the school or camp bus. We wait in other places like motor vehicle agencies, restaurants, hair salons, automobile repair places for oil changes and such, doctor offices, department stores, post offices, and train stations. We wait on the phone for customer service issues. When we go out with family, we at times have to wait for family members to exit a public rest room. Sometimes you have to wait on a long line for the rest room, especially if you are a woman! We sometimes have to wait for a table at a restaurant. If we bowl, we have to wait for the other bowlers to finish up before we can get an available lane. We sit in the bleachers and watch our children play sports. I am sure you can share some of these experiences and even come up with other places that suck up so much of our time. In the meantime, we either stand or sit there - waiting. The waiting is collectively longer than we think. After some internet research, I found that in an average lifetime, the total time we wait in lines ranges to about two to three years. For some of us, I am sure that time is even longer, depending on our lifestyle. Why not make the waiting a productive use of time? We can certainly use that waiting time to get in better shape. I have come up with a way to get my exercise time in so I can be productive while I wait, without looking ridiculous!

I can only imagine what some of you are thinking. You can picture me doing jumping jacks or something embarrassing in public? Well, no, not really! The exercises I do are very discreet and people do not know that I am exercising at all. It looks like I am a little fidgety, but it is not noticeable by most.

I do a combination of toe lifts or heel lifts. The heel lift is when you raise up on your toes and your heels are raised. You can hold the pose on your toes for a few seconds. You could also do the heel lifts at a slow and steady pace. I then switch to toe lifts, where I rock on my heels, lifting my toes up. I try not to hold this pose too long, in fear of falling back and hitting the unlucky soul who is behind me in line. Sometimes I alternate, doing a heel lift, and then a toe lift. All are done slowly and trust me, do not look ridiculous! It just looks like I am rocking back and forth, like many who are waiting in line. Holding my stomach in while doing this is another added benefit.

Another way we waste time is waiting on the phone while at home. We are put on hold while we wait to speak to a human being. This includes calls for bill inquiries, repairs, catalogue orders, and such. Calls from friends, relatives, and businessmen also take up our time. How do we handle these kinds of calls? Most of us sit idle while handling these calls. Some choose to stand. There are some who will do chores while on hold, which is at least a way to get things done and get some kind of exercise in. We can also do more exercises while waiting. We can even be more adventurous, especially since we are not in public and can feel free to move around more. For those who sit or stand, these exercises are for you!

While holding the phone (or even putting the call on speaker phone), stand and do side leg lifts. Stand on one leg, putting a bit more weight on this standing leg. With the other leg, do a side lift, moving it out to the side in controlled movements. Again, books and even the internet have great instructional photos and videos. Instead of counting in your head, which could be a distraction from an active call, time a minute per side, alternating. Do a minute of side leg lifts on the right side, then the left. I also like to do leg lifts, but to the back. Instead of lifting the leg to the side, I am holding it behind me and kicking backwards. Squats or half squats are helpful as well. There are so many exercises that can be done while waiting on a call or even taking a call. Feel free to do sit-ups, jumping jacks, or exercises targeting an area you feel you really need to work on. Instead of sitting, get up and do some exercises! For more ideas, do a search on the internet or find an exercise book that has doable exercises you can handle. This is an excellent way to get in the exercise, making unproductive time very productive.

You can also get in exercise while talking to friends, associates, and colleagues. I can get in exercise without thinking about it and focusing completely on the speaker and our conversation. Sometimes people will stop me at the gym to chat. Sometimes I run into good friends when I pick up my son from school. Other times I run into people at a public place and a conversation ensues. While standing, do some of those exercises. The main exercises I do during these conversations are heel lifts or toe lifts. I do not have to count them, which makes it easier to pay attention to the person who is speaking to me. No one suspects that I am exercising. It is very discreet, yet very productive and beneficial overall.

Another way we waste time waiting is watching our children play. It is not a waste to watch your children, just a waste to not be active along with them. I oftentimes see parents standing around on the playground, watching their children swing, slide, run, and jump. Some will gossip with another parent on a park bench and watch their children. Instead of watching your child play on a playground or even at home, why not get in on the action? Get involved, even if it is for ten minutes. Play a game of catch. Bending to catch the ball alone is a great form of exercise. Get in that pool and swim with your child. Do not watch from the sidelines. Play a game of basketball or soccer. Just kicking the ball around for a few minutes is a good form of exercise. You will feel youthful and you get to burn calories too. Your child will also enjoy the quality time you are giving. If your child is older and no longer thinks parents are cool, either play parallel to them, not with them, or ask them to "deal" for a lousy ten minutes. If attending a child's sport, don't sit on the bleachers or in that comfy folding chair. Get up and do some heel or toe lifts. Be more adventurous in public if you dare!

CHAPTER 18

How to Handle Stress

*L*ife throws a lot of things our way. One of these things is stress. Unfortunately stress knows no boundaries and can occur inside and outside of the home. A response to such pressures is to fill ourselves with something. Because of the pain we are going through, whether emotional or physical, we want to take in something to feel better, to be fulfilled. Some turn to alcohol for comfort. For others, it is drugs. For the many people like us, our drug is the food.

I used to utilize food to medicate myself in any type of stress. For example, one of the main treats I would eat in times of stress would be a whole pint of fattening ice cream. I easily convinced myself that it was the right thing to do. After all, I went through a stressful day; I deserved a nice treat. If it was not the ice cream, then it was the chips, doughnuts, muffins, candy, and other fattening "niceties." As I was eating, it felt great, but the aftermath was not worth it; I felt stuffed, weighed down, and sick. Additionally, weight was easily gained as a result of taking my "medicine." Guilt and self hatred followed as a result of doing such a foolish thing. Unfortunately the cycle repeated. As stress seeped in, so did all the fat, calories, and misery.

If we must fill ourselves with something, it has to be the right thing. We have to fill ourselves with things to get that long - lasting, ultimate satisfaction. I equate this concept with a swimming pool. You fill the pool with what it needs - water. You fill it directly, ensuring the hose of running water goes directly into the pool in order to fill it. Moreover, you are filling it with what it needs, as opposed to filling it with mud and rocks. Therefore, fill yourself with what you need instead of junky, fattening food - the mud/ rocks.

What do I do to fill me up when stress comes my way? I do so many things. I will gladly share a portion of these things. I am sure you can come up with good ones on your own!

- Meditation - Taking time to relax is soothing.
- Bath - buy fancy bubble bath that is reserved for de - stressing times.
- Make time to do something fun to reward yourself (besides eating).
- Put on music that makes you happy.
- Call that special someone who you can vent to and who can put a smile on your face.
- If food is a must, grab something healthy. See the chapter on Munchies Disease for ideas. Munchies Disease is a term I give when the desire to grab garbage food is immense.

I would like to highlight the importance of meditation. This way of handling stress is so helpful. Did you ever feel like a string of events is caving in on you? Nothing seems to be going right and you receive aggravation in stereo. As you know, the old person I used to be would grab for the ice cream or chocolate. Feeding a broken heart was one of the things I did best. The new Lori meditates. Do not bring excuses into the mix such as not finding the time and the space. Everyone can spare three to five minutes, and everyone could pick a small space (vacant room, car, closet). If all other plans fail, there is always the bathroom. If it is the only quiet spot you can find, use it! Choose the best position and close your eyes. If you sit criss cross and hold your hands out as people do in yoga meditation, do that. Just sitting with eyes closed does wonders. It is a form of release that increases calmness and decreases the desire to medicate ourselves with food.

A possible added bonus to meditating is sleeping better. For some, meditating makes for a better night's sleep. The body is more relaxed and sleep is more peaceful. There is less exhaustion, a factor that can cause overeating. I cannot tell you how many times I would eat for the soul reason of being tired and not thinking it through. Sometimes I would eat for the sole purpose of waking myself up, getting more energy. This involved consuming sugary foods. The foods I chose never did help me gain more energy, but that did not stop me from trying time and time again.

So if you feel pressure, do not run for the snacks and other goodies. Run to meditate so you can calm your body, mind, and soul.

Whether it is meditation or doing something else to make you feel good, do it without reaching for the bad food. Unfortunately problems hit us so many times, and to respond to such stress by overeating will guarantee certain failure. We need to program ourselves to react differently to stress. Though life is challenging, food will not make us happy and it will not solve our problems in the end. In fact, food could cause more problems, compounding the stress.

CHAPTER 19

How to Handle "Failure"

You ate more than you should have at the party. You overdid it at the gathering in your own home where you had more control of your food. You had a grandiose case of the Munchies Disease and snacked on everything in your view. You let a food pusher have his or her way with you, leading your "willpowerless" self to eat something fattening. You overdid it at a restaurant. You got more than a little carried away between Christmas and New Year's Day. You were out of control with eating while on vacation. The bottom line is that you ate more than you should have. The result is weight gain, and perhaps an overstuffed feeling that day and the next, or both. What do you do?

The old me would quit immediately. Negative feelings surged, which resulted in beating myself up inside:

"You are a failure and you can't do anything right. You have no control. Just give it up because you won't succeed anyway. You failed just like you did all these years trying to diet."

And I would give up, eating more and more each day until I gained back the weight I lost and then some. It was a formula for failure. I "fell off the wagon," beat myself up emotionally, and returned to awful eating habits. The new me, however, handles these "failures" differently. I put quotes around the word "failure" because deviating once in awhile is not a true failure. To me, failure is something permanent. A binge fest or any slip up that leads to weight gain is not a permanent thing that will hinder you from your goals. The weight gain is fixable and is not going to stay on you forever, unless you do something about it. This is what you must keep in mind. Straying from healthy eating is not a sin. We are human. The undesired results are fixable. We can make up for it, but we have to take immediate action. (We can't have an occurrence and say it is okay, but do the same thing the next day and the next.) Make the "mistake," but fix it right away.

One time when I had company over, I was disappointed to find a two pound weight gain the day after. This surprised me greatly; I thought I burned a lot of calories cleaning like a fiend prior to our guests' arrival. I ran around serving all evening, burning even more calories. My food choices were healthy. It was disappointing to say the least. I must have had more food than I thought. Out of all honesty (as always), it could have been partly due to my upcoming period. I always tend to gain weight during that time. Regardless, it was a two pound gain no matter how I looked at it. The old me would have berated myself and would give up altogether. The new me "said" inside my soul:

I'm not happy with the weight gain. I'm not exactly sure what happened, but I know how to fix it.

I went to the gym the next day to, as I call it, "work off my sin." I use the word "sin," playfully. I certainly did not do something abominable. What I did was do something that is okay, natural, and fixable. I managed to lose the weight within two days and was back on track.

One time I went out to lunch with a friend of mine. We dined at an Indian restaurant. I'm a multi - cultural eater and absolutely love Indian food. Needless to say, I really delved into the food and stuffed myself. I had that weighted down feeling. Waking up the next day, I found myself sluggish and stuffed. The old me would hate myself. My conscience would convince me that as a result of this over eating episode, I cannot succeed and will never succeed in losing weight - ever. The new me with the new attitude/approach thought differently. I couldn't wait to go to the gym that morning to work it off. My positive spirit took over, as I vowed to travel further on the elliptical machine. My drive was strong and failure did not exist. After exercising, I actually felt better and was not sluggish.

One Thanksgiving holiday season was extremely memorable. On the special day, I made sure to make the meal in between lunch and dinner time, around two in the afternoon. That would afford me more calories if I had two meals combined. I was careful, but was able to still enjoy my favorite foods. I took smaller portions and did great…until the next day. We went to movies with a friend and her son. We then went to lunch, and again, there was success in my eating. Later on it was dinner time. I decided to make some of the Thanksgiving leftovers. You know what they say, some leftovers taste better than when they were first cooked. I let loose and ate more than I should have. The old me would have beaten myself up and quit any kind of healthy eating. Instead, I took a "stock check" on how I felt. Overeating made me feel bloated. I could feel my stomach stretched. I was weak and fatigued. This reminded me of the 272 pound me. This is how I felt most days because I overindulged so often. Therefore, the new, thinner me made myself really take note of how I felt. This was something I did not want to experience again. It was enough for me to forgive myself and strive to not let it happen again, or even often. Thereafter, I tried to remember that awful, stuffed feeling that sapped the strength out of me. I did work out at the gym the next day, not feeling bad in the slightest. I realized I was human and should not be scrutinized. I realized I did not want that awful feeling again, and knew it would revisit if I kept up that way of eating.

Prior to these episodes, I had plenty of pitfalls. As written previously, I gained weight while on a cruise. I also gained weight after one of my knee surgeries. I had to walk with a cane for weeks and could not get around much. Once I could solidly stand on two feet, I got on the scale and to my horror, saw the 20 pound weight gain. Part of me wanted to quit, but I stayed true to my new attitude and pushed forward to lose that weight. I did, and continued on my journey to losing over 100 pounds. Regardless of our pitfalls, it is important to get back on track.

The bottom line is to not quit if there is a "relapse." Do not give up at all. Gather up your positive spirit and press onward, not dwelling on what you did wrong. Plan for the future on what you are going to do right! So if you gained two pounds, so what? Lose three next time, slow and steady!

CHAPTER 20

What to do to Keep the Pounds Down and Motivation Up

As you lose weight and as you reach your goal, you need tools to keep the weight down and your spirits up. It is so easy for motivation to decrease. So many things trigger quitting or relapse. Stress and challenges make us stray from our goals. We have to make sure we have defenses to battle such problems that come our way.

Keep Your "Before" Pictures

Let's say you are about to walk into a restaurant, party or any even that has a lot of fattening foods. What do you do to keep from straying? Carry your old photos of your heavy self. In my purse, there is a small plastic bag with four pictures of me at my heaviest. I look at them good and hard, asking myself, "Do I want to go back to this?" I continue my inner conversation. "This is what you have to go back to if you don't behave. Do you want to go back huffing and puffing again? Do you want to go back to big, loud clothes? Then behave yourself!" Putting such pictures on the refrigerator helps too.

Medicate Yourself With Anything But Food

Problems will come your way, unfortunately. That is a major part of our lives. Such things may make us want to grab for the candy or mass quantities of food. Instead, treat yourself to non food items. If you have the money, get a massage, manicure, and/or pedicure. Say to yourself, "Gee, I have been through hell, I need a _____!" (Insert a non food item in the blank.) Go for a walk to blow off steam. Purchase clothes or shoes you always wanted. Soak in the tub. Purchase that piece of technology you always wanted. You know the things, both large and small, that will make you smile. Don't turn to food as solace for your troubles. Instead, turn to pampering or simply doing something nice for yourself. Most people do not feel this way because deep down they feel that they do not have true self worth. We must change this negative way of thinking and be kinder to ourselves.

The People Who Build You Up Are the Same Who Tear You Down

Think of all the hard work you put into weight loss. People start to notice and send many compliments your way. Think about what they will all say if you gain it all back. Sure we should stand tall and not care what others think. In this instance, we should truly care what others say - it will "scare" us into not gaining the weight back.

Let's look at my situation. I lost over 100 pounds. My friends, family, and clients noticed. Employees and members of my old gym complimented me hundreds of times combined. In my third year of my healthy lifestyle, I received more compliments that year than in my entire lifetime. Additionally, the gym did a feature story in their newsletter about my weight loss success. Additional articles appeared in newspapers, a magazine, and on the internet.

People have approached me and told me I was a hero. Others

said I inspired them. I recently found out from my hairdresser that someone from the gym raved about me and said that she admires me. She also added that I am the reason for her weight loss. My hairdresser knew it was me right away.

What if I gained all that weight back? What message would I send people? Would that message be that they really can't lose weight and keep it off? That they can't achieve a healthy lifestyle? I would be just like everyone else. I once read that about 95% of people who lose weight gain it all back within a year. Taking off the weight and then putting it on is a far too familiar dance we do. Did I really want to show failure, just like "everybody else?" Or, did I want to inspire, showing that if I can succeed, anyone can.

What are the other repercussions for gaining weight? There would be laughter and disgust. I would be gossip fodder, where people would gather and laugh about my failures. I can almost hear them now...

"Did you see how much weight she gained? She's *huge!*"

"Ugh, she came so far and then let herself go like that. Man!"

People love to see others fail, especially when it is at something they have trouble doing themselves. It makes them feel so much better to see that others can't succeed as well. People love to talk about such failures. This shows that they can't do it either, which is a comfort to them. As mentioned previously, that is why tabloids have a "Look Who Got Fat" section for those celebrities who gained weight. Of course they show the picture of the once svelte celebrity next to the current picture of the heavier soul. People love this type of article, which is why magazines continually showcase it. The public loves the rise and fall, enjoying the failure of somebody else.

Though I was never one to care what others think (during my adult years), I use this to help keep me on track. I also do not want to invalidate my articles; reporters took great care in writing about my success story. I did not want such a story to become a major failure. I do not want to be a joke, a laughing stock. I want to be a role model for others and show that anyone can do this, succeeding overall and not failing. The aftermath of such failures of the past keeps me on track. I do not want to slip - it would be a long, painful fall.

Put Pictures Up of An Outfit You Want to Reward Yourself With

As I was losing weight, oftentimes I would see a wonderful outfit in a catalogue, but knew I was not yet at a size where I would look good in it or even fit into it. I knew I had to work towards this goal to wear this outfit. I would post the picture on the refrigerator and wrote *Go for it!* beside it. This fueled me to push forward so I could someday wear something similar. Even a picture of a thin, not anorexic looking model, could help increase motivation.

Put Post-its Up That are Filled With Compliments

In an earlier chapter, I mentioned to write down compliments you receive and post them on your mirror. These little morale boosters will keep your spirits up and you will remain on the right track. Do what is more meaningful to you. Either write it on a post-it or small piece of paper yourself or ask the person to write it for you. Explain that these words are so special and you would love to have them as a keepsake and morale booster. Read them from time to time and understand how highly people think of you. Read those encouraging words! Such positive statements give us the motivation and strength to carry on!

Get Revenge on Your "Enemies"

Though I am not a vengeful person, I like to show off to people who insulted me and did not believe in me at all. For me, it feels good to show people who doubted my abilities (time and time again) that I could actually reach my goals without their "support." I also enjoy showing off to those who have ridiculed me because of my weight.

A family member made a comment that I gained soooo much weight since my wedding. A couple of family members would sing to me, "I don't want her, you can have her, she's too fat for me!" They enjoyed the tears they caused. An obese coworker (who weighed less than I did back then) made snide comments about my weight gain after viewing a wedding picture on my desk. Well, I am thinner than all of these people now and wear a smaller pants size than them! Many people commented to be cruel, but some who have insulted me in the past had more of the insert foot in mouth syndrome, saying things without thinking. Please note that this is not a competition. I do not size myself up against people to determine who is "thinner." I simply take note of only those who insulted me and what these people look like now. Regardless of the personality types, it feels good to be thinner than those who made insensitive comments. Looking better than the "tormentors" can give a great deal of satisfaction.

Several "friends" did not give me support at all. Hey, I would have been glad if they did not say anything and simply allowed me pursue a healthy lifestyle. Unfortunately there they were, the naysayers who told me that I am just going to fail again like everyone else. I am thinner than some of them. Some are just so thin with their tiny frames that I will never be as thin as they are. It does not matter, though. I did reach my goal and I did not fail as they predicted. Succeeding despite doubts is truly great "revenge" for those who were incredibly unkind.

An ex-boyfriend's mother told me that I will be overweight for the rest of my life. She said I will always be heavy like her daughter -in- law. This was not said in spite. I was dating her son at the time, and things were good between us. She thought this comment was helpful, but it was not. The sticks and stones saying is not true. Words do hurt and I had that carried around in my heart. I remembered it as my yo-yo diets failed. Now I get to prove her wrong, another thing that makes me happy and gives me another type of "revenge." Of course I do not wish anything bad to happen to her. It just gives me great satisfaction to disprove this woman's prediction and I succeeded in spite of what she said.

Though this should not be the major reason to lose weight, it could be a small part of the reason. Prove these negative people wrong. Show that you can succeed, despite their predictions.

Take Up An Activity/Hobby/Sport That Will Get You in Great Shape

Taking up an activity that you have done long ago, or not at all could help you feel youthful and determined to get/stay in shape. For me, that activity was dancing. I used to dance when I was a child, and gave it up to concentrate on college studies. After 23 years, I decided to take an adult tap class. It was very exciting. I did not jiggle as much when I danced. I found I was better at it than originally perceived, regardless of the 23 year gap. Dancing made me feel so youthful, so energetic. When the dance recital costume came, I tried it on, becoming more determined to lose weight so I can look fabulous for recital photos and the recital itself. The recital photos looked great. I even took some photos with my son and loved how they turned out. I didn't look overweight at all and even looked a few years younger. When the recital time came, I got up there without any nervousness traveling through me. I had complete confidence. My husband later remarked that I looked really happy dancing on stage…and I was! It was so much fun! Dancing lessons keep me in check, for I want to look good for the pictures and for myself. When I get onstage for all to see, I want to make sure I look presentable.

There are many dance classes, exercise classes, and even sports teams at all age levels to participate in. For instance, a local college has an adult volleyball team that is open for all adults to try. Some towns have a recreational department that has sports for all ages. So take up something that is both good exercise and is good for keeping your body in check.

Keep Progress Pictures In View

As you progress, take pictures of yourself. This will show that you are a winner, succeeding in what you are trying. Keep them in view so it reminds you not to stray. I have my dancing pictures in my kitchen prominently displayed. I like the way I look in these photos, and make sure I look at them to keep me on track.

Kick Away Negative Thoughts and Excuses

Oftentimes a negative thought or excuse will pop up. This occurs in my life regardless of how much I try to maintain a positive spirit. Remember that negative thoughts and excuses are leading causes of failure in anything people strive for. Try not to allow your mind to complete these thoughts or excuses. Kick it away and think of something else. At the very least, kick it away and counter it with something positive.

Home Luggage

...for home sweet home...

CHAPTER 21

Get Rid of Putrid Diet Food and Hide the Culprits!

The title of the chapter says it all. It is important to do some "spring cleaning," of the food in your home. Get rid of the bad stuff and hide the tempting culprits! Most people will not fight me if I tell them to get rid of terrible tasting food. This chapter tells you what to get rid of; omit diet products that taste disgusting! I believe some of you are thinking, "I'm with you!" Most of us have tried reduced fat, no fat, and reduced calories and fat products. The trouble is that some are absolutely atrocious! There was a time where most of my purchased food was "dietetic." The salad dressing was too acidic and putrid. I remember forcing myself to eat the salad, cringing as I tasted this gross chemical concoction. The diet cheeses I tried were either tasteless or were equivalent to offal. The texture was also different compared to regular cheeses. Instead of a smooth, moist piece of cheese, it was rough and dried out; this was its normal texture! Many diet cheeses reminded me of thinly sliced rectangles of wax! Certain diet entrees were inedible. The diet ricotta and cottage cheeses were awful and unfulfilling. Such disappointments in taste and texture are enough to make dieters quit.

I must be clear and say some diet food is amazing. Food

companies have made great efforts in making these alternatives to the high calorie versions. However, there are many products out there that have come my way that make it unbearable to eat or even look at.

My advice is that if you found one of the "good" diet foods, feel free to use it. Make sure it doesn't contain carcinogenic chemicals, substances that could cause cancer. I tend to migrate towards the more regular foods and take a natural approach most of the time. If I want a cookie, I will not eat the one that tastes like cardboard just because it is low in calories and fat. I will have the regular cookie that tastes great, and I just simply incorporate it into my diet. I will end up satisfied instead of disappointed. To me, it is better to eat one "good," fattening cookie than a calorie and fat equivalent of five disgusting, cardboard tasting diet cookies! Disappointing foods like these make us quit the fight to eat right. So do not avoid your favorite foods. Make them work into your diet without going over on your calories and fat. And stop suffering with the awful tasting "diet food."

Now that we got rid of the putrid food, is important to hide the tempting foods, especially when we get that Munchies Disease, grabbing food that is in view. One of the culprits that help us fail in our mission to lose weight is the fatty food lying around the house. Many homes showcase a vast array of hard candies and wrapped chocolates in bowls that are found in living rooms and family rooms! Sure, most will claim this is for guests, the company. We all know too well that the residents of the home reach for the goodies too. The tall, attractive cookie jar is right on the kitchen counter within easy reach. Clear cookie jars are worse, where a victim walks by and is lured by the sight of the treasures inside. Clear glass containers store chocolates and other goodies. Let us not forget the bowl of nuts; a handful yields major grams of fat. The old me would not just walk by and pass up goodies. I had to take a handful of something, and convinced myself that it is only a "little bit." I was obviously fooling myself. Food addicts rarely take a little bit. Handfuls of this and handfuls of that can only hurt our journey to healthy eating.

Most kitchens nowadays have an island for food prep. Whether I am visiting or whether I am going to a home for tutoring, I almost always see tempting foods on the island. This is an area that is passed by often and is in the best view for grabbing. In my home, I try to keep the good stuff out of plain view.

I have a husband and son who like a good cookie once in awhile. I do not want to deprive them. Therefore, all treats should be placed somewhere that is out of plain view and is out of a major foot traffic area. Possibilities of good storage areas include cabinets, drawers, closed pantries, or a special tote bag in a closet. Goodies in plain view make a person want to grab for them again and again and again...

There were times where I felt that I was not going to eat anything. I was not hungry and I did not feel like consuming a thing. Then I would see that bag of cider doughnuts that I bought from the farm the other day. Seeing that and other tempting treats made me convince myself that I was hungry and I had to fulfill my need. Many calories and several grams of fat later, I ate food I did not need. I certainly ate food that my waistline did not need!

Hopefully out of sight would indeed mean the high calorie, high fat entities are out of your mind!

CHAPTER 22

Munchies Disease, Late Night Snack Attacks, and Brushing

This is a disease that hits us all unexpectedly, primarily in the home. We come home from work or errands and just have to grab food and pop it in our mouths. Sometimes it can strike at work when we see the dreaded candy dish or food put out for some kind of celebration. We could even be at home for awhile and then the urge hits us. We must eat something and fast. This disease also occurs when stress hits us. As a result, we <u>must</u> have a lot of awful food to kill the pain! In the previous chapter, we learned to keep tempting food out of sight so we do not grab for it in passing. However, with Munchies Disease, we will grab for what we see and even raid areas where food is concealed. It is a desperate attempt to grab something, and fast! Usually what we snatch is not the healthiest for us. Nuts, chips, chocolate, and ice cream are the favorites for us to grab. I get Munchies Disease often. There is no cure for it. I have to eat something, so I thought of ways to pop food in my mouth that won't cost me my waistline.

One of my foods that I love to pop is frozen fruit. I get the crunch and sweetness, which is so satisfying. I will wash red grapes and put some in the freezer. They crunch very well. I do love frozen cherries that are sold in the supermarkets. These are pitted and are not saturated in syrup. They are all natural, crunchy on the outside, and slightly soft on the inside. They are not as hard as the grapes. Frozen raspberries are another favorite of mine. One thing to be mindful of is the kind of teeth and mouth sensitivity you have. Some people get tooth pain when eating something extremely cold. Some people cannot chew hard things like frozen fruit. If you find it difficult to chew, thaw the portioned fruit for about five minutes and test it to see if it is "chewable" for you. Another method for a quick thaw is running the frozen fruit under lukewarm water.

Another thing you can do is portion out a snack like pretzels, crackers, or chips and put each portion in a small plastic bag. Do this ahead of time so you are unlikely to cheat and take more than you should. A good tip is to brush your teeth before divvying up the snacks. Be sure to set aside the bags in a special place. One bag per day, please! Do not eat four small bags of snacks. That of course defeats the purpose! These snacks can be for those Munchies Disease emergencies.

Most salsas are good to have for a snack. Most are zero grams of fat and have very few calories. For instance, one of my favorite salsas, a mango and peach, has 25 calories and zero grams of fat for one tablespoon. Sometimes salsas are a "free food" on some diet plans. This means a person can have it without limits. I will grab a handful of baby carrots, and will carefully cut each lengthwise. This gives the carrot a flat surface so more salsa can pile on top of it. Carrot sticks work as well. Try not to use tortilla chips. If so, measure out a small amount, depending on the calories and fat the chips pack. Truthfully, I have found that when I pile salsa on a chip, I can barely taste the chip anyway; the salsa taste overpowers it. Carrots are nice and crunchy as well, and are a great low calorie substitute for the high calorie, high fat chips.

Another food to grab quickly to satisfy is the tomato! No, I am not talking about an everyday tomato. I am talking about a special type that a friend of mine got me hooked on. They do go by many names but are golden orange cherry tomatoes. They are unique because they are incredibly sweet. They are bursting with sweetness and are crisp, making them very satisfying for a snack or any type of craving.

Popcorn without butter is very satisfying. There is less fat, and a less greasy feeling when delving into the bowl. Because of my dislike for that grease on my fingers, I avoid microwave popcorn altogether. I invested in a popcorn popper and love to make freshly popped popcorn. I spray the top with either butter flavored cooking spray or pump olive oil buttery spray, and then season it with a powdered cheese. It is magnificent, and tastes good fresh and when eaten later. I oftentimes make some ahead of time and still enjoy it. At times I buy a bag of kettle corn, which is reasonable in the amounts of calories and fat. I have a small bowl that fills a cup and a half of it if filled to the rim. Therefore, no measuring is involved. I just pour and eat. Try not to dig into the bag to grab some. Dump into a small bowl like mine and enjoy. If you do not have bowl, dump it into a measuring cup and even eat it out of this cup. No fanciness is needed to enjoy a snack.

Sometimes I get the "Munchies" when I am preparing dinner. I am so hungry, and handling food makes me desire food more. It then seems difficult to wait twenty minutes or so to wait until dinner is cooked. My old mindset made me grab for any bag of chips or candy I could to tide me over until dinner is ready. The new Lori reaches for grapes or raspberries instead. I throw some of this rinsed fruit in a small bowl and pick at it as I prepare dinner. This satisfies me until dinner is ready.

Most people seize something as soon as they return home from work or an errand. A way to eliminate or curb the "disease" is to drink a full (eight to ten ounces) bottle of spring water ten minutes before arriving home. This will make you feel fuller and less likely to indulge as much or even at all!

Munchies Disease can grow rampantly, but if it does come upon us we can be prepared with the antidote to cure it or curb it. We can easily choose good foods that won't expand our waistline!

Late night snack attacks were not so much a problem for me as it is for my friends and relatives. It is a form of late night Munchies Disease. People feel they just have to eat something at night. My husband for instance, put on pounds just for late night snacking. Meals were sensible throughout the day; the one to two hours before bedtime were challenging for him. He felt he <u>had</u> to eat something and choose chips, nuts, and pretzels. Snacks were by the handful, and even by the bowlful!

My friends snack as my husband did, but some put more effort into the snacking experience. One friend of mine would automatically get up at midnight and fix herself a sausage, peppers, egg, and cheese concoction. One would eat sandwiches at night. Another would eat a mountain of cereal with milk. Another friend would eat leftovers from that night or the night before. You do not have to be a nutritionist to know that these snacks are high in calories and fat, causing significant weight gain if such eating rituals continue. Most of us are less active at night, so lounging around will not burn off calories and fat. Going to bed on a full stomach doesn't help either. It also does not feel so good while lying in bed. The morning after does not feel great as well. Many wake up with that weighed down feeling.

My advice is simple - do not eat at night! Make dinner your last meal, and incorporate this solid rule into your life. Most who snack at night are so used to this ritual that they do not consider how bad it is for them. Many eat when they are not hungry. It is timing that calls them to the food, not true hunger. It is time to eat, that magic time that is always reserved for snacking, hungry or not. Most see nothing wrong in a "little snack" which would lead to more calories and fat than they perceived.

Depending on how voracious you are for late night snacking, eliminating it altogether can lead to significant weight loss. That weighed down feeling will be gone during the night and when you wake up. There will be a better feeling both inside and out when food is not weighing you down. Even if you start weaning your way off of the habit, having less and less for that late night snack, it would be a plus. A drastic cutback will not yield success. Have less and less food at night and soon you will not miss it!

For me, the disease hit when I prepared food or cleared plates. These are healthy lifestyle "crumblers," impeding chances of eating right. When I would make a peanut butter sandwich for my son's lunch, I would help myself to two heaping spoons of peanut butter before proceeding with the preparation of his sandwich. Placing snacks and desserts in sandwich bags was also a problem. More chips, crackers, and the like would end up in my mouth than in the sandwich bag. If I was baking cookies for a bake sale, I would pop a nice handful of chocolate chips before putting any in the batter. If I was preparing a meal with cheese, I would eat a few pieces of the cheese before using it for the main dish.

A trick I use is to brush my teeth before making a lunch, going to a supermarket with food samples, preparing a food, or before cleaning the dishes from our meal. Feel free to brush before doing other things that may lead to binge eating. From experience, peanut butter and the minty toothpaste taste do not go well together. The mint flavor makes the peanut butter taste awful. Chocolate tastes atrocious in this combination as well. In fact, most foods taste bad right after brushing. Brush whenever you feel like. It could be before making a meal, making someone's lunch, clearing plates, or even if you have a simple craving. Another trick is to bring mouthwash on your travels. You can even bring mouthwash or toothpaste to work and use it just before stepping into the workplace area that is filled with the temptations. If you have a craving, rinse your mouth. I tend to want to munch on something after working out. Before leaving the gym, I rinse my mouth with mouthwash so I do not grab for a snack. Try this! You will soon have a smaller new you and a sensational smile!

CHAPTER 23

For Good Measure

One way we lie to ourselves is with our food portions. We eyeball the amount and assume we are correct in our estimations. The bottom line is that our eyes lie to us. We take more than we should. Regardless of measuring the same amount on the daily basis, we can stray from that amount if we stop measuring.

I have been measuring my food for five years in a row. I did a little experiment one day. There is a hot oat bran cereal that I have very often, cutting up different fruits to put in it. I usually measure out ⅓ of a cup of this cereal, which, when water is added, cooks/puffs up to a hearty hot cereal. I tried to simply pour the cereal into the bowl, eyeballing the ⅓ of a cup. After pouring the cereal into the bowl, I poured the cereal into a measuring cup to see if I was correct in my estimation. I was way off; I poured ½ of a cup. This amount may seem minute, but picture over measuring foods that are high in calories and/or fat (but still can be good for you). What if you measured twice as much of peanut butter or almond butter? How about sugar, butter, or margarine? What if we measured too much of that? For various foods and ingredients, it does indeed make a difference.

If I had a choice of using a measuring cup or a food scale, I would opt for the scale. There are very cheap scales out there for purchase and are so well worth it. A cup of cereal for instance could be a heaping cup of cereal if not leveled. Weighed food would not be leveled with the measuring cup and a more accurate amount can be attained. Nutritional labels give the serving sizes in tablespoons/cups and grams/ounces. Weighing the serving size will help get a better handle on portion control.

Sometimes rushing around and being tired lead to not wanting to take that one extra step to measure food. We do not feel like weighing or getting out measuring spoons or cups. Regardless of how we feel, regardless of how rushed we are, still grasp a measuring tool and use it. It will not take as long as you think and will be so worth it. If you do not do it, expect to take more than you should. I have been lax in measuring with other diets. The weight would pile on and I would wonder why. I would then sense failure and quit.

Regardless of how many times you have poured a specific amount, do not convince yourself that you do not need a measuring cup or measuring spoon. You do need it. I need it, and I am always measuring. Perhaps you can make a good approximation, but over time the eyes get greedy and the amounts creep up to more than what was wanted. So invest in a scale, a measuring cup and measuring spoons. If you are on vacation and your accommodations include a kitchen of some sort, bring measuring utensils along. If bringing food to work, however, I would pre measure and put it in a container/storage bag.

Measuring at home can actually help you for quantifying food at a restaurant. Let's say you want to have a 4 ounce portion of cooked chicken. Weigh four ounces of the cooked portion at home. Use an object you will definitely bring to a restaurant and utilize that for size comparison. For instance, half the size of your wallet or the full size of your change purse may be close to the size of four ounces. A compact mirror may be close to the size of the portion. Perhaps a credit card/identification card could be helpful. Once you identify an object to compare to, use this in the restaurant to determine appropriate portion. This is a way to approximate portion sizes and keep control.

Another way to measure is by using a standard spoon. We all know a standard spoon size restaurants have. It is one of the larger size spoons. Use a soup spoon at home and request one at the restaurant for more accurate measure. At home, use this spoon to measure non heaping spoons of rice, for instance. If you are looking to have a serving size of a cup, see how many spoons it takes to fill a measuring cup of rice. If it takes, let's say 8 spoons, then at a restaurant, use 8 spoons to get the right portion size and set the rest aside to take home or simply leave on the plate. You will have these values in your head or you can write it down and put it in your wallet/purse to refer to. After awhile, it will become second nature and you will not have to think about it.

Regardless of how we feel or regardless of the excuses we have, grab a measuring utensil and quantify!

CHAPTER 24

The Candy Holidays

There are plenty of holidays for candy. That means plenty of opportunities for failure, especially in the home. Such days include Halloween, Valentine's Day, Easter, Mother's Day, birthdays, Thanksgiving, Christmas, and even New Year's. The failure is not restricted to those days. The candy lasts for many days, even weeks, giving even more opportunities for failure.

For me, Halloween is hell for many reasons. I do not excuse or support vandalism on Mischief Night or any other night. It is a shame when some children visit for candy and lack good manners. These factors alone make me the Scrooge of Halloween. Another reason to grimace over Halloween is the candy. The old me had no control. I would give out three pieces and eat five! This pattern continued and I would get so sick and overstuffed. When I used to shop for Halloween candy, I would buy what I loved to eat. It is a natural thing that we all do. We certainly do not buy candy we hate - we buy what is more appealing. So I grabbed for the bags of the delectable goodies that tempted me the most. After all, why shop for awful, disgusting candy when the favorites are more tantalizing?

The trick is to buy candy that is unappealing to you. This sounds obvious, but we are on automatic pilot, purchasing what we like to eat, what is indeed great tasting to us. The new me purchases candy I loathe. Therefore, I will not eat it at any time. I can give it out to the children without even being tempted to dig into the bowl. Therefore, purchase candy that you do not enjoy. I personally purchase something that is not chocolate, since chocolate is so tempting to me. Find your most "unfavorite" candy and give it out on Halloween night. Most likely you will not delve into candy that is not one of the favorites. If you feel you must have a treat for yourself, either brush your teeth, keep yourself busy, or set aside one single serving size bag of popcorn or pretzels, making sure you give out the rest. If that is too tempting, do not prepare a treat for yourself and just focus on giving out the candy you hate to the little ones!

A question many people ask me is how I handle the candy that my son brings into the house. Let's face it, he does not mainly bring home candy I detest. There are lots of my favorites in his candy bag. The solution I have is to not even look at it. In this day and age, it is important for adults to check the candy for tampering. That is my husband's role. My son knows to take his candy into another part of the house and not even show it to me. My husband checks it and my son is allowed three pieces a day until he finishes or until he gets sick of it and allows the rest to rot in the bag. (The latter is usually the case. Two months later I end up throwing out his stash.) If you have children who go out to collect candy on Halloween, instruct them to not show you the candy when they return. Let someone responsible check the candy, and allow them eat it in another room so the temptation is not there. As an aside, restrict their candy intake as well. If lots of candy is not healthy for you, it certainly is unhealthy for your kids. If you feel better checking the candy or have no other option, have your child show you a few pieces he or she wants to eat at that time. Rinse your mouth with mouthwash before looking at the candy! Sometimes it is difficult to watch others enjoy candy. As an aside, whatever you do, please do not allow your children to eat candy in a room alone. Choking is a possibility and you want everyone to be safe! If someone else cannot be present in the room, be there, but busy yourself with something else while in that room, not directly looking at the "candy fest" your child/ children is/are enjoying.

Candy gifts are the worst because it is not the gift of your choosing. Of course it is a common practice for birthdays, Valentine's Day, Easter, Mother's Day, Christmas, and the like. People present a box of these goodies to you and then you are stuck with it. Some friends and relatives of mine have me puzzled in this area. Many of them knew I was trying to lose weight. Most know of the struggles with temptation in the quest to lose weight. Therefore, why in the world did they choose candy as the gift of choice? Would anyone purchase a bottle of wine for an alcoholic? Why buy candy for a person who has difficulty in controlling quantities of food? (Keep this in mind for those who are in the same situation. Use that money to buy a gift card instead.)

Regardless of my feelings, I would graciously accept the candy. I was grateful for the gift, but would then give it away to a friend who can handle the candy sensibly. Some people can control themselves, and/or do not have a weight issue, so I would give the gifts to these people. I would not regift - that I detest. I would give them the candy as a bonus. For some, I would kindly ask them to take the candy off of my hands, and they would gladly oblige. Another great idea is placing it in the faculty room of your child's school. True every school is different, but there are a lot of schools similar to the one my son attends. I tutor in the teacher's lounge and oftentimes I find goodies on the table. I am sure they would appreciate a sealed box of chocolates they can open up and enjoy. If you cannot find someone worthy of this candy, simply toss it in the garbage can on the road in a public place. Then you cannot rethink your decision when you decide there is a need to break open the box. When it is tossed, it is gone! Another option if you cannot get out is opening the box, dumping the treats into the garbage. Make sure to pour some kind of wet garbage on top of it in case there is a change of heart and you end up fishing for them in the trash can! Do not worry about wasting candy or money. It was not your money that was spent on it, so throw it away without the guilt.

For those you can really talk to, explain that you would be truly grateful if gifts were not edible. My husband does know not to give me a heart shaped box of chocolates for Valentine's Day. He knows candy, cookies, and other treats cannot be gifts for any holiday. That is the open communication that we have. People I cannot speak freely to are my clients. Sometimes I do not know if they are even going to buy me a gift for the Christmas season. It would be tacky to tell them what to not buy me. Therefore, I accept the gifts graciously and dispose of them quickly. If I know I have the strength inside me to resist, I will bring the gifted candy box around to my students as I visit for sessions and allow them to enjoy the delicacies. This is a nice treat for my students and they are thankful. Although candy is a huge part of the gifts I receive, I am still grateful for their generosity. It is indeed the thought that is most important.

It does take a lot of strength to get rid of treats that we absolutely love. Keep in mind that it is for a good cause - you! You are a good cause and are certainly worth it. Think of all the calories and fat you are saving. Find other ways to celebrate an occasion without tearing through a gift box of delectable goodies.

CHAPTER 25

Isolate Your Food, Not Yourself

One thing you must be sure to do is not isolate yourself. You do not want to serve something "really delicious" to your family while you chew on a carrot. Include yourself as well; just make the meal du jour a lot healthier.

I never cook overly fatty foods, but sometimes my husband's and son's favorites are a little too high in calories and fat for me. If I make macaroni and cheese, I cook the pasta and then isolate my portion in a separate bowl. In the pot, I put the amount of cheese they enjoy. Again, it is not a tremendous amount of cheese, but it is too rich in calories and fat for my eating lifestyle. I then put a slice of cheese on my portion and microwave it until the cheese melts. That amount of cheese is truly satisfying, and I can enjoy the same meal with my family.

Another favorite of mine is cheddar mashed potatoes. This is an easy and savory recipe. Boil small creamer potatoes until soft. Mash in the pot with a potato masher. Add skim milk. At this point, I need to isolate my portion. I put it in a small bowl or mini soufflé cup. I add one slice of cheddar cheese on my portion and microwave it for a brief time. I then add the appropriate amount of cheese to the remainder of the potatoes so my family can enjoy.

I must admit that I rarely use low fat or zero fat cheese. As mentioned in the *Get Rid of Putrid Diet* Food chapter, most taste awful and are not satisfying. They also contain extra chemicals to compensate for the taste that is lost when the fat is reduced or completely missing. I want to enjoy my food and do not want to deprive myself. How unsatisfying it is to suffer with disgusting diet cheese in macaroni and cheese. The bad taste would make me reach for something else. I also want to eat foods that are more natural and not have added chemicals in them. True regular cheese contains more fat and calories, but I budget into my diet. I will not use three slices. One broken in pieces and melted in macaroni and cheese or even in mashed potatoes is far more satisfying than awful tasting diet cheese in larger quantities.

Another meal that I make differently for myself compared to the rest of my family is pizza bagels. I do cook the pizza bagels together, but will make sure I know which one will be mine. I put less sauce and cheese on my portion and put generous amounts of these ingredients for everyone else. If there is room for confusion, I will simply cook mine in a small pan.

Sometimes I serve an amazing avocado cheese dip on an average day or even at a gathering I host. I put two tablespoons of it in a small bowl for myself. This avoids dipping pita chips into massive amounts of dip. I would have no idea how much I am scooping. I could probably scoop a tablespoon of this amazing dip per chip. The tablespoons add up, and the dip is not dietetic. By isolating my portion, I am able to still enjoy without taking in the massive amounts of calories and fat.

I make a hearty soup to die for while my husband and son have ground beef with cheese. I use a lean ground beef and cook it with a little garlic powder and onion powder. I cook mini shells pasta and put the beef on top of the pasta with a little sauce and grated cheese. I pull two ounces of ground beef and two tablespoons of shells and put it in one cup of prepared tomato soup that I heated for myself.

This makes a hearty tomato soup and I get to have the same food my husband and son have. True I can have the exact same dish in a healthy portion size, but this is another way to get variety in foods.

You can still have that cake and eat it too...just not in huge amounts. Separating portions is a good tool that will help you reach your weight loss goals. It also makes everyone happy. You can have a satisfying food without overindulging while others can have the freedom to indulge! Of course, take care of your family...they can indulge, but not too much. They need to be healthy too!

CHAPTER 26

Recipe Renovation

There are a lot of amazing foods I would like to try. When it came down to the recipe, I would discount it if it had too many "fatty" ingredients. For instance, a waffle recipe called for four tablespoons of butter! Another recipe called for two sticks of butter! The old me would crumple the recipe and throw it in the garbage. The new me utilized my chemist skills. I began questioning quantities and ended up modifying a plethora of recipes that still taste great with such modifications!

What would happen if I cut the amount of butter/sugar in half? What if I substitute this lower fat ingredient?

After major changes, the food I prepared would turn out to be fantastic. I cut butter, margarine, and sugar amounts in half. I have substituted heavy cream with a 50/50 skim milk/heavy cream mixture. Cutting back or substituting just the right ingredients in just the right amounts can make a recipe delicious and healthier.

Here are some ideas for reductions/substitutions:

- cut the sugar for chocolate chip cookie recipes by half or even by 25%. These recipes call for white and brown sugar, so there will be a lot of sugar to begin with. The chocolate chips have sugar which also contributes to the sweetness, thus reducing the need for extra sugar.

- cut butter/margarine in half. If the food does not taste great as a result, cut it by 25% instead. When I experimented, I found I did not miss the butter at all when I cut the amount in half.

- use applesauce in place of oil. A friend of mine used this substitute for a muffin recipe. I was the official sampler, and I have to say that it tasted sensational! The recipe certainly did not need the oil.

- use Greek yogurt instead of oil or butter. I do direct substitution. For example, if the recipe calls for ¼ cup of oil, then I will use ¼ cup of Greek yogurt. Though yogurt tastes sour, it goes undetected in such recipes in which it is not one of the base ingredients.

- cut the amount of oil in half. I have done that in the past and did not miss it.

- never grease the pan. Some recipes call for greasing the pan with butter or margarine. Of course that adds a great deal of calories and fat. Use a nonstick cooking spray, which works just as well.

- cut back on the amount of chocolate chips the recipe calls for. Sometimes there are too many chocolate chips in the batter. If you are a chocoholic and love your chocolate chips, cut it by at least ¼ of what the recipe calls for. If the recipe calls for one cup of chocolate chips, add ¾ instead. Cutting back a little really helps a lot...and you won't miss those extra calories and fat grams!

- use light mayonnaise instead of oil, even if it is for a cake! One day at a restaurant I ordered a piece of chocolate cake for my husband and me to share. The server proudly commented that the chocolate cake is moist. After a bite, I wholeheartedly concurred.

"You want to know the secret ingredient for that?" he asked. "It's mayonnaise."

After learning that, I tried mayonnaise in cakes and it does add a moist texture. No one can taste the mayonnaise at all. So as ridiculous as it may seem, experiment with the mayonnaise, especially light mayonnaise.

Try to be a chemist in your kitchen and replace fattening, high calorie ingredients with healthier, low calorie ones. If your confidence wanes, there are a series of cookbooks that incorporate a lot of these healthy ingredients. Sometimes vegetables are added and you can never taste them. Before grimacing at the spinach that is used for a muffin recipe, for example, try it. You will be surprised that you cannot taste the vegetable. These recipes also taste great so you get taste satisfaction and a healthier alternative.

I am currently placing the finishing touches on a cookbook that has a variety of recipes. Such are inspired by many cultures to give variety. My collection consists of low calorie, low fat creations that taste great. I utilized my chemistry skills to experiment and substitute. For instance, in a rice pudding recipe, I substituted a corn starch mixture to get the desired creaminess instead of using heavy cream. The taste is amazing. Ingredients are natural and do not include sugar substitutes. One popular cookbook for "healthy cooking" incorporated so many sugar substitutes and other chemical concoctions. This was abominable! So hopefully I can present to you a cookbook packed with snacks, appetizers, soups, main meals, and desserts. I made major recipe renovations, but the end result is a great recipe collection. To ensure such, I gave food samples and questionnaires for every recipe I made. If ratings were stellar for recipes, they were included in the book.

We are oftentimes focused on sticking to the recipe that we do not even consider changing things here and there. So try reducing those ingredients and you can start reducing you!

CHAPTER 27

Bulk Up Your Desserts and Even Some Main Meals

You can indeed have your cake and eat it too, but realistically, portion sizes have to be smaller. We cannot dole out a huge slab of cake or two cups of ice cream and expect us not to gain weight, especially if this ritual is done a few times a week. There is no way to reach our goals by eating mass quantities of sugar, calories, fat...

We can make things a little better to increase our satisfaction. A scoop/half a cup of ice cream looks kind of lonely and unsatisfying. A good way to fool our eyes and satisfy our taste buds at the same time is to bulk up our desserts the healthy way.

What do I do to my lonely scoop of vanilla or chocolate ice cream? I add frozen, unsweetened cherries. If you experiment and target the right brand that has good, naturally sweet cherries, you will be in "heaven." You may have to shop around at a few supermarkets to find them; I found two brands with decent frozen cherries. Even a health food supermarket carries frozen cherries, so do the research. Add one half of a cup of frozen cherries and mix it in the ice cream. The scoop looks bigger and the ice cream tastes wonderful. Be creative and try other unsweetened fruits.

Fresh is also acceptable but I sometimes like the frosty crunch the frozen fruit brings to the ice cream. If you have sensitive teeth or are not crazy about hard, frozen fruit, opt for fresh. If the frozen fruit is tough to chew, thaw it or go directly to fresh fruit. Make sure all frozen fruits used have no added sugar, corn syrup, or other sweeteners. Go for the natural stuff! Here are some combinations I have tried with both fresh and frozen fruits that I added in my ice cream:

- cherries
- raspberries
- raspberries and peaches (best in vanilla ice cream)
- peaches
- blueberry/raspberry/blackberry combination
- mango slices
- strawberries
- strawberries and raspberries

I am sure that some of you can come up with great concoctions in addition to these. Keep in mind that additions must be low in calories and fat. For instance, do not mix in a load of chocolate chips. Five chocolate chips on top as a small garnish would be acceptable. And do not talk yourself into having hot fudge or caramel sauce as a topping. I used to convince myself that these toppings were an absolute must, and would pour enough to make a hot fudge or caramel swimming pool for my ice cream to float in. The ice cream is sweet enough, so try to avoid them and go for the more natural ingredients.

At the time of this writing, there are a lot of ice cream parlors in my area that have self serve ice cream. This involves dispensing your own soft serve and toppings. The cup of your ice cream sundae creation is then brought to a scale and weighed. You are paying by weight. What I do in this situation is I use the bulking up method. I get frozen yogurt that has low calories and fat. This information is usually located on a sign above the frozen yogurt dispenser. I put a small amount of the yogurt (I try to eyeball a half a cup) and then bulk it up with lots of fruit. These places have a lot of fruit choices: raspberries, pineapple, blueberries, mango, strawberries. These are fresh, not the processed, syrupy kind. I make sure to load up on the fruit. My sundae looks amazing and huge. It looks satisfying and I do not feel deprived in the end.

Breakfasts can be bulked up with fruit as well. Oatmeal tastes great with a little milk and fruit. I put a half a cup of strawberries, raspberries, cherries, or peaches in my oatmeal. These fruits are also good in a hot oat bran cereal. I sometimes put a half a cup of vanilla almond milk into the hot mix and one of the fruits mentioned. Cold cereals could benefit from fruit as well. Try it out. Depending on the cereal, certain fruits will be great additions while others will not.

It is also important to note that you can bulk up some of your main courses too. A salad with simple vegetables, especially the non starchy ones, could be less satisfying. This could make hunger come way before the next mealtime. What I do to bulk up my salad and feel visually and physically satisfied is to add ½ cup of chick peas (garbanzo beans) or cannellini beans. Such additions make the salad appear very robust. The beans fill me along with the rest of the salad and I feel more full.

Garbanzo or cannellini beans are very good additions to soups. There is a creamy tomato basil type of soup that I buy from time to time. Heating one cup of this soup in the oven with these beans yields a tastier soup with more volume. Additionally, I will wash and throw in baby spinach leaves about five minutes before the soup is finished cooking. Try this, even if you are not a spinach fan. The creamy tomato flavor is absorbed into the spinach, and the leaves do not have that typical spinach flavor. This bulks up the soup and helps you get the proper nutrition. I also like eating soup that has solids in it (e.g. crackers, rice, chicken, beef), as opposed to a plain liquid, so this is ideal for me. I love this combination and feel full.

Adding pita chips to certain soups can also be great. Limit the pita chips to about ten or twelve. Experiment with soups and chips to see if the combination is to your liking.

Another main meal that I bulk up is the chicken kabob. I marinate the chicken in a special marinade (e.g. teriyaki, honey Dijon, lemon garlic) or purchase the chicken that is already in a marinade. I use kitchen shears to cut the chicken. I skewer the pieces of chicken, but put "bulking up" pieces in between. I put slices of red pepper, Vidalia onion, and mushrooms in between. By the time I am done, my four ounces of chicken on a skewer looks pretty huge with all the pepper, onion, and mushroom pieces that are in between. And it is filling too! Sometimes I bulk it up so much, that I divide the four ounces of chicken into two skewers. It then looks like a large amount and looks filling and satisfying.

Pizza is another food I bulk up. There is a chapter dedicated to pizza, but it is worth mentioning here. Oftentimes I make pizza using a medium to large tortilla. I put sauce and a quarter cup of shredded cheese. I then bulk it up like crazy! I add mushrooms, onions, and broccoli. It is very pleasing to the eye. It looks large and that big pizza is all for me!

Be an experimenter. Let your kitchen be your laboratory and explore amazing and creative combinations. You may surprise yourself on what you create! So create and look great!

CHAPTER 28

Lunsserts

When I was a child, I loved making up words. It was not that I wanted to make up a new language. I came up with little words to express my feelings. I used the words "bestest" and "trafficky." One word I am purposely creating today is "lunssert." This is a cross between lunch and dessert. It is a main dish that is a lunch and a dessert all in one. It can collectively have fewer calories and fat that having a main dish and a dessert separately. I have several ideas for lunsserts that can contribute more flavor and fewer calories and fat...and it is oh, so satisfying!

I make a great Greek yogurt lunssert. I tend to favor Greek yogurt because of its taste and thick texture. I measure ¾ of a cup (0% or 2% fat) and then cut up one to two kinds of fruit. Some people like it "syrupy" as is found in yogurt products with fruit on the bottom. In this case, I would pulse the fresh fruit in the blender, then add it to the yogurt. Well cut cherries, raspberries, blueberries, or peaches are great additions. If I want something a little more substantial, I will add one cup of either Special K, mini shredded wheat squares, Rice Chex, or Honey Nut Cheerios cereal on top. Feel free to experiment with other cereals! If I take this meal to go, I put the cereal in a separate container and add it just before I eat the yogurt mixture. If I add it ahead of time, the cereal gets soggy in the yogurt. This combination is a tasty meal; I get the sweetness of a dessert and the crunch of a snack. It is very satisfying and it stops my craving for dessert. I get my main meal and dessert all rolled up into one!

Another lunssert would be three tablespoons of low fat ricotta cheese. In this case, do not opt for the non fat ricotta cheese. All I have tried tasted terrible! One cup of cut up fruit on top of it makes a great lunssert. It is very satisfying. The cup of fruit can be of one kind or mixed. It is delicious and filling. Fresh fruit is best, but frozen fruit can be a great substitution.

Lunsserts are great if there are time constraints. On one occasion for example, my errands took longer than usual. Someone stopped me on my way out of the gym. Of course that took extra time. Afterwards, I ran into a friend of mine at the supermarket. That also took longer than usual. By the time I came home and put the groceries away, it was soon time to get to my next tutoring appointment. Instead of getting fast food en route to the appointment, I threw together a quick lunssert. It was the Greek yogurt with peaches. I cut up a few cherries and put a cup of Special K on top. I got the crunch of the cereal and the sweetness of the fruit, which were satisfying. I was able to have a meal in the small time frame that I had.

Another lunssert favorite of mine is the French Toast recipe below. It could be a breakfast item, but it makes a great lunch entrée. The fresh fruit adds to the sweetness, making it a great dessert part of the meal. To get the maximum flavor, use fresh pineapple and fresh cherries. Use a pineapple corer to avoid pineapple hassle!

Loni's Pineapple French Toast Lunssert
(serves 2 to 3, depending on size bread used)

Place two pineapple rings and ½ cup cut cherries in a preheated pan treated with nonstick cooking spray. Let that cook over medium, turning occasionally for even cooking while blender ingredients are prepared.

Ingredients for blender:

- 1 large egg (white plus yolk)
- 1 large egg white
- 2 fresh pineapple rings
- 2 teaspoons of cinnamon/sugar blend
- 1 tsp vanilla

Put all ingredients in blender and blend until smooth. Place mixture in a wide enough bowl where bread can lay in mixture evenly and will not curl up in a bowl. Dip bread, preferably wheat bread, whole grain into the mixture for about 5 to 10 seconds each side. Having the bread sit in the mixture longer will make it soggy and will fall apart. Place in a preheated pan that was sprayed with nonstick butter spray. Put bread in pan and flip when cooked on one side. Size of bread will vary cooking time on each side.

Serve with cooked pineapple/cherry mixture on the top of the bread or on the side.

Open Faced Baked Cheese and Blueberry Bash! (serves 1)

I got this idea while shopping at one of my favorite grocery stores. Normally I bypass free samples, but this combination intrigued me: blueberries and cheese. Surprisingly, it makes an amazing combination. The sample was actually a blueberry spread on a small slice of cheese. I thought it would be better tasting if I incorporated fresh blueberries instead.

Ingredients

- 1 slice of whole wheat bread (a good tasting kind!)
- ½ cup blueberries (raspberries work just as well if you are not in a blueberry mood)
- 1 slice muenster cheese

Preheat oven to 350. Spray a cookie sheet with nonstick spray. Put a slice of bread on the sheet. Top it with one slice of cheese and berries. Put in the oven and bake 15 minutes. The cheese should be melted and the bread should be nice and crisp. For a crispier top, broil for one to two minutes after baking.

Ravishing Ricotta Berry Blend

Add ½ cup of either cut strawberries, blueberries, raspberries, or mangoes to the blender and pulse five quick times.

Add to ¼ cup of ricotta cheese and mix.

Drizzle with honey and a light sprinkle of cinnamon if desired.

With a little creative chemistry of your own, you can make your own concoctions. It is a great alternative to have from time to time. It is satisfying and convenient, especially when there are time constraints. Most often a quick meal is not a good quality meal. These lunsserts are very tasty, satisfying, and healthy. It is also great to have while on the road or at work. These are quick, easy, and healthy! Who could ask for anything more?

CHAPTER 29

Popcorn Palooza!

Popcorn is a great to curb the Munchies disease and it makes a great dessert as well. One of the many useful items I have invested in is a popcorn popper, a wise alternative to microwave popcorn. Even in my obese years I hated dipping my hand into a bag of microwave popcorn and pulling up popcorn and grease. I hated the way my hands felt and I knew if it didn't feel good in my hands, it certainly did not do any good in my body.

The popper that I bought is the kind that has a lid which serves as a bowl. The popcorn is amazing! I only add one teaspoon of oil for the popping. The popcorn tastes great without any topping. It tastes better and is obviously fresher than store bought bags. If I do want to explore with a topping from time to time, I select a "butter/ cheese" concoction. It is easy and flavorful. Spray the popcorn with butter flavored cooking spray or with an olive oil butter spray (found in the dairy aisle). Sprinkle one tablespoon of grated cheese on top. My favorite is parmesan cheese or a mix of grated parmesan and Romano cheeses. The cooking/butter spray wets the popcorn so the seasonings can stick to it. There are many other seasonings to experiment with: Cajun seasoning, cinnamon, et cetera. Be a scientist - experiment!

As mentioned in a previous chapter, *Stop the Shoveling and the Stuffing*, it is important to eat food slowly. Sometimes that is a challenge when it comes to popcorn. It can be difficult to eat one kernel at a time. There could be a desire to grab handfuls. Ideas were shared in the chapter on how to control eating mass quantities at once, but some ideas here are exclusive to popcorn! If the urge is to grab, use a small spoon. We use a spoon for cereal, don't we? Why not use a spoon to eat popcorn? For a greater and more fun challenge, why not try eating popcorn with chopsticks. That utensil will surely slow down eating! Doing such things will help you enjoy the delicious popcorn, one kernel at a time!

CHAPTER 30

Pack Smart or Pack on the Pounds

So many people make excuses for eating out. I am talking about reasons that are not social. Dining out becomes a need where people want to frequent restaurants, sandwich shops, fast food joints, cafeterias, and the like. Here is a list of my past excuses:

- *I'm on the road. I have to eat out somewhere.*
- *I am in the workplace, so I have to eat in the cafeteria or order out.*
- *I'm too busy in the morning to make lunch. Buying a meal is faster and more convenient.*

This is a whole lot of nonsense, of course. The truth is we want to eat that fatty food. We do not feel like making food, fussing and planning. It is so much easier to purchase a meal because it is fast and tasty. We feel like treating ourselves. We all deserve a treat, but it is the frequent treating that becomes the problem. Unfortunately most choices are unwise and we end up packing on the pounds instead of simply packing a meal.

As I mentioned in the beginning of this book, my job had me on the road quite a bit. I had a tall stack of take - out menus in my glove compartment. Depending on where I was, I pulled out a menu for my favorite place in that area and phoned ahead. I would enter the eatery with the satisfaction of knowing the food was ready for me to gobble down. I would then quickly devour it as I hurried to my next appointment. My selections were never wise, never healthy. Choices included stacked hoagie sandwiches, ravioli, eggplant parmigiana, chicken parmiagiana, burgers, pizza, and chicken in some kind of cream sauce. At times desserts accompanied my selections: cannolis, rice pudding, cake, doughnuts. cookies.

My eating during corporate life was also poor. When I was not traveling, I was eating in the cafeteria. Again, my selections were poor. Meat or chicken in some sort of cream sauce was chosen. Tall sandwiches with lots of mayonnaise, along with massive desserts were eagerly placed on the tray. Some of us would go out to lunch from time to time. The group I was with always loved to order a bunch of appetizers and then share. In addition to the fatty entrée, I had lots of greasy appetizers to devour!

What was my solution to this eating frenzy? It was to drop the aforementioned excuses and make an effort to pack a decent lunch. I tackled my three primary excuses:

I'm on the road. I have to eat out somewhere.

Yes, I am on the go, but I don't have to eat out. I can make my own lunch and do not have to rely on an eatery. I could prepare my lunch the morning of my travel or the night before. I can make it work and it isn't an absolute must to purchase fatty food.

I am in the workplace, so I have to eat in the cafeteria or order out.

No, I don't. I can buy a large insulated lunch bag and put a variety of foods in it, from something small like sandwiches to something large like a plastic container of salad. Add an ice pack or two, and it will last all day. The lunch travels with me and is easy to grab when I have a free moment.

I am too busy in the morning to make a lunch. Buying a meal is faster.

If time is an issue in the morning, I can pack the lunch five minutes before bed after brushing my teeth. Brushing my teeth does not make me crave food as I am handling it. Then in the morning, the lunch bag is in the refrigerator, all set to go.

Here are some of the things I pack in my lunch. Hopefully you can try some of the main meal options that are "doable," whether a microwave oven is within reach or not.

- 2 slices of whole wheat bread with one level tablespoon of peanut butter. In a small container, keep sliced strawberries, raspberries, or blackberries. Add fruit to the sandwich just before eating.

- Salad (already prepared lettuce mix) with a variety of vegetables (tomatoes, zucchini, peppers, onions, celery, et cetera) with ¼ to ½ cup of chick peas (garbanzo beans), ¼ cup dried cherries, and 1 tablespoon of feta cheese. In a small container, put 2 ½ tablespoons of dressing (dressing sticks to the sides of the container so after pouring it you will have a nice, solid two tablespoons of dressing). Add dressing to salad just before eating or else the salad gets soggy when you are ready to eat it.

I like salad dressing with more taste for fewer calories. My current favorite is Trader Joe's Champagne Pear Vinaigrette dressing. Two tablespoons only had 45 calories and 2.5 grams of fat! There is a lot of flavor to this dressing without having to ingest lots of calories and fat! A lot of the ginger dressings are flavorful, with few calories and fat.

- Pita Pizza
  - ○ Small to medium whole wheat pita. Put two tablespoons of sauce, three tablespoons of shredded mozzarella. Separately grill vegetables that you enjoy (not in oil) and place as a topping. Bake at 350° for fifteen minutes. Let it cool. Wrap in plastic or put in a microwaveable container. Eat cold or put in a microwave oven and cook for about 30 seconds.
- 4 ounces ground beef or burger, cooked. Cool and then crumble in a salad with two tablespoons of dressing.
- Strawberry soup
  - ○ One cup of nonfat or lowfat plain yogurt
  - ○ One cup of strawberries
  - ○ ¼ cup orange juice
  - ○ 1 tbsp sugar
  - ○ ¼ cup water
  - ○ pinch of cardamom

Put all ingredients in a blender. Puree. Chill and serve. This travels nicely when put in the correct container. This is an excellent main course and dessert all rolled up into one! Another Lunssert!

For more elaborate lunches on the go, cook a little extra for dinner so you have leftovers for lunch. You could simultaneously cook dinner and your next day's lunch at the same time. This type of organization and planning ensures that you have a healthy, decent meal. My beverage of choice for these lunches is always water. For a little pizzazz in your water, add a lemon or orange slice, and let it sit in the water for hours. The juices seep into the water, making it a tasty beverage.

I still like a good dessert, so I make sure to pack something decent. I include one of the following in my lunch bag:

- sandwich bag full of grapes
- cup of cut strawberries/raspberries
- one cup honey wheat pretzels
- one cup of kettle corn (this snack has the crunchiness, saltiness and sweetness that I crave)
- two tablespoons of dried fruit and nut mix
- one large honeycrisp apple
- one chocolate biscotti
- two seedless tangerines

Packing smart starts at home, so pack wisely, strategically, so overindulging does not occur.

CHAPTER 31

Snowed In? Snow Problem!

Most of us, whether we live in hot or cold climates, have been restricted to our homes. This comes in forms of hurricanes, snow storms, and the like. When we have no choice but to be cooped up in our homes, you know what that means…we have more time to eat! We are also more confined, which means we are closer to the "good" food; this leads to stronger temptation. Additionally, being snowed in means that there is nowhere else to go and most of our homes are not large enough to move around in them much. This obviously makes it difficult to get in a good cardiovascular workout. Moreover, not all of us have exercise machines in our households! If you are like the old me, you would eat out of boredom, sadness, and overall frustration while being restricted to the home.

Perhaps some of you feel "house entrapment" is a rare occurrence, but where I live it happens more frequently. Living on the east coast, I had to deal with Hurricane Irene, snowstorms, and more recently, Hurricane Sandy. There were plenty of opportunities to stay shut up inside and to pig out. The latter hurricane became more challenging, for we had lost power and there was a major gas shortage. There was nowhere to go because other businesses were closed. Additionally, roads were blocked with fallen trees and other debris. Gas was limited so it was not wise to venture out anyway.

One radio station reported that people who were shut in from Hurricane Sandy were most likely to gain ten to fifteen pounds. I did not fit the bill; I did not gain a pound because I came up with a system to keep me eating and exercising right.

Food portions did not change. The key is to stay out of the kitchen between meals. Being there triggers the desire to eat. I did not want to see the tempting foods that I had. This would cause me to eat more than usual. Activities were directed anywhere else besides the kitchen. I also made sure to put away foods from the countertops to make sure I did not see it. As the old saying goes, out of sight, out of mind.

I made up a slew of activities to do. When the power was out, I used my iPod to play tunes. My husband, son, and I had a dance party. Each of us got to pick a song and we all danced to it; this burned a lot of calories. We reserved this activity for the daytime so we would not bump into each other at night. We played catch with balls that were indoor - friendly, so as not to break anything inside. I would do sit ups or exercises I remembered from my exercise videos whilst my husband and son played one - on - one soccer with the indoor-friendly ball. There were free weights, a set of five pound dumbbells, which were well used that time. We also played board games, which took my mind off of snacking. This went on for almost a week, but I did not falter. Keeping busy was what prevented me from raiding the pantry.

A common response to being cooped up is to have "pity parties." These "woe is me" rants in our minds prevent us from eating healthy. Pity surrounds our inability to get out, possible/definite damage to our house and property, and/or the dreaded clean up after the bad weather passes. Whatever the defeated reason, people tend to eat, utilizing food as a medication. Recognizing the pity party as soon as it begins and then putting an end to it can really make a difference.

Some naysayers may ask why I would go through an entire chapter to try to prevent a pigging out that would last a day or two. The answer is that some of these crashes, even if for a day, could cause individuals to give up completely. Most would say, "I give up. There is no way I can control myself so I might as well stop my efforts." Getting through this challenge gives one a sense of pride and it gives that individual strength to continue eating right.

Luggage You Need For Venturing Out

(This section covers all aspects of venturing out, not just vacations!)

CHAPTER 32

Park the Car Far

You may have heard this time and time again, especially in January under weight loss New Year's Resolution Tips. Park the car farther when frequenting a supermarket, mall, or shopping center. Do not take the closest spot. If you have a disability and cannot do this, you are excused! For the rest of us, do it! NO excuses! Every little bit of exercise counts, especially because most of us say we do not have enough time to exercise! Therefore, get it in when you can, and this is a perfect opportunity!

For some of us, we need a little bit of motivation to do something like this. After all, there are excuses of fatigue, lack of time (need to get in and out of the store), and temperature (too hot, too cold to walk a little further). We can certainly spare an extra minute to walk to and from a store. In short, it is not as bad as you think. Well, how about a little reality to up that motivation and eliminate excuses. I proudly present to you problems that come with parking the car close to a store or mall:

People slam their car doors into your car...and guess what?

What is the answer to the above? It is simple - most people do not care if they slam their doors into other cars! You should have seen all the dings and scratches my old car had. Sure, some marks were from rocks and snow/ice. Most came from the ignorant and inconsiderate. I have seen people fling open their car doors and hit cars, including mine while I was sitting in my car! Let's face it, this is a selfish world that we live in and people just do not have consideration for others. Parking far eliminates the chances of cars parking close to yours. Most cars parked furthest have no "company" and can remain there with little chance of dings and scratches.

The shopping carts go wild!

Carts seem to move around the parking lot aimlessly without anyone guiding them. This is due to wind and people not caring about the carts staying in place after they take the items out of them. As a result, carts slam into parked cars, causing even more damage to the bodywork. Most carts are aggregated in the front of the parking lot and are rarely clustered in the back of the lot. Therefore, park the car far so there is less of a chance of a cart slamming into your vehicle.

People block your side so you cannot open your car door.

In close spots, there is more activity from neighboring cars. People are going in and out. Some have their side car doors open as they stash groceries and other items. Some have a stroller in the way which blocks car entry. An individual for instance, does notice that the driver of a neighboring car wants to enter or exit his or her vehicle. Do they care? No! Most do not even hustle just a little bit to accommodate. Individuals refuse to move their doors in just a little to make room. Some just leave their car doors open and do some mindless activities. The bottom line is that people do not make room for others, so parking away from the busy part of the parking lot will eliminate this problem.

When you park further away, think of all the benefits you will have aside from getting a few seconds more of exercise. There will not be as much crowd activity. No one will block you from entering or exiting. Car doors will not fly open and strollers will no longer be obstacles. Carts will rarely ram into your car. All the activity will occur toward the front of the lot where everyone wants to park because it is closer. If you park far, you will have less parking aggravations, a reduced ding/scratched car, and more exercise!

I was never one to get a fancy car. My mom told me when I got my first new car that it is wonderful, but it should be viewed as a machine to get me places. If there are dings and scratches, I should not aggravate myself. This was my mentality and all cars were simple, bottom of the line. My most recent car was no different. After 125,000 miles in four years, it was time to get a new car. I was going to get the lowest model of a particular car. To make a long story short, the dealer had to get that model from another dealership. After two weeks of waiting patiently, they went to pick up the car, only to find out that they sold my car out of greed! Angry, I asked for a refund. Words were exchanged and deals were offered. To appease me, I got the top of them line car for the same price! This has the "bells and whistles." It is sportier looking and is the nicest car I ever owned. I take care of the car, but not too crazy. I do not wash constantly and try to clean every spot or splash. I do park the car far away in the lot and so enjoy it. I get to walk a little further and I do not have to worry about people blocking me or slamming car doors into mine. I feel less suffocated and can move around freely. I do not have to make room for someone entering or exiting a spot; no one comes near me. It makes life easier and I do get the extra benefit of extra walking time. My car also received less dings, but could not avoid a major dent when a deer ran into the side of it! At least such damage did not result from parking the car close!

Parking Far Can Make it Easy to Get out of a Spot

How many times do we want to pull out of a spot and encounter so many obstacles? People stand alongside your car, making it difficult to back out. The clueless pedestrians walk in front of your car. Some stand too close to your car to chat with others. Kids are allowed to wander aimlessly as well. Other cars back out, blocking your ability to leave. The possibilities go on. About 90% of those problems dissipate if the car is parked away from the cluster of cars and people.

You Most Likely Will Find Your Car Faster

Which row? Which spot? Depending upon the layout of a parking lot, it may be easier to find your car if it is apart from all the others. In most lots, I never have to second guess myself. I see my car all alone in the back of the lot.

Does it sound like I am giving strategies for parking in shopping centers? Am I digressing in my old age? Well, no, not really. I am trying to motivate you to find ways to get more exercise into your life. Walking a minute more is progress. Outlining additional benefits justifies the idea of parking the car far. In the busy lives we lead, it is important to get exercise in any way we can. This includes while waiting in line (thus the chapter *Lose Weight While You Wait*) and when we need to park our cars.

So have an open heart and try this! Parking the car even a little further away from the shops reduces aggravation and increases calorie burn!

CHAPTER 33

Can You Gross Yourself Out While You Are Out?

The "spit" birthday cake mentioned in the *Party of Fat in and Out of Your Home* chapter is a good introduction for this "grossing out" theme. Remember people blowing out the candles, getting their spit all over the icing? Remember how some families allow the children to take turns to blow out the candles, yielding more spit? Thinking about these gross factors works for some people, including me. Such thoughts make the food very unappetizing. Take a look at that food, really look at that food. Make sure you are analyzing the food that is the fattening or "bad food." Pay attention to detail; what you see may make you not want to eat it.

Let's visualize that birthday cake scene. People sing "Happy Birthday" and the birthday person blows out the candles. There are germs being deposited on the cake, which you will "enjoy" after it is soon served to you. Do you really want to eat spit cake?

Building on that, how about that person who serves the cake? I cannot tell you how many times I saw a person serving cake, licking his or her fingers every time icing got on them, which is often. After licking the fingers, the person then proceeds to serve more cake, touching every piece to ensure proper placement on the plate. Now you have the spit of the birthday person and of the server. Are those added bonuses you really want?

The chips, pretzels, candy, and other treats in bowls make it tempting. But think of those people with dirty, unwashed hands, delving into the bowls. How many times have we seen people leave a stall in a public rest room and NOT wash their hands? Picture the germy sick person coughing into his hand, then reaching for a treat that you will reach for later. What about sneezing and coughing near the bowls of food? How about that relative who just changed her daughter's dirty diaper in the car just before walking in and does not wash her hands! How about that double dipper who dips a chip in a dip, bites into it, and dips into it again with the contaminated chip? Unbeknownst to you, there will be germs on your food. That is enough to deter you from even sampling the contaminated food.

Another grossing out factor are greasy hands. Some snack foods such as chips are so greasy, that your hands will feel grimy after reaching for that. Do you really want that grease and grime in your body? I sure don't; it grosses me out.

Sometimes I visit doughnut shops to purchase a cup of coffee. At most of these places, the smell of doughnuts permeates the air. It makes me want to buy a doughnut to accompany my cup of coffee. However, when I look at the bins that hold these doughnuts, I see big, greasy rings of where doughnuts used to be. These doughnuts are so greasy, that grease actually leeches from them onto the wax paper they are resting on. Removing a doughnut reveals a circular stain, which looks disgusting. Do I really want to put that blob of grease into my system? There is a huge ring of grease where the doughnut used to be, so imagine the amount of grease that is still left in the doughnut!

Another grease trail can be seen after buying cookies. When I used to purchase cookies, they were put in the bag. By the time I brought them to my home or whatever destination, there would be spots of grease on the bag. It was disgusting!

Picture yourself in a fast food restaurant. To some, the greasy smell is a turnoff. To some, they think, "Yum!" Hopefully you can use that smell to your advantage, getting repulsed by it. Most fast food kitchens are open, where consumers can see almost every aspect of the food preparation. We can see the workers taking the metal basket of fries out of the fryer. Did you notice all the grease that drips out from the fries once the basket is raised? You know there is plenty of grease in those fries. The fries are so saturated with oil that it drips off of them. You will be ingesting plenty of it. Does that look appetizing to you?

That dripping oil is the very same that seeps through the bags for takeout fast food. One time after hosting Bingo at the assisted living center we normally volunteer at, my son and I saw a family bring in a couple of bags of fast food. From a distance not within earshot of the family, I pointed out the grease blotches to my son. That really grossed him out. Now it is another reason why he will not eat greasy food. Grease is just not attractive or the least bit appetizing.

I cross reference this in the upcoming *Supermarket Frenzy* chapter, but gross yourself out when you pass by free samples. Some of these samples are left in a bowl or on a plate for people to sample freely. I try to think back to how I saw people take these kinds of samples in the past. Some cough near the samples, readily spreading germs on the samples. Some cough into their hands before dipping their germy hands into the food. Think of those who frequent the public rest room and do not wash their hands. These and others who touch filthy things are also digging into these sample foods, contributing more germs and bacteria. Do you really want these free food samples now?

How about that creamy soup you bought at a takeout place? You had some extra that was not eaten, and you put it in the refrigerator. When you take it out to eat it the next day, it is a glob of lard. It solidified into a grease glob of fat! A lot of fatty soups congeal like that; it is a liquid when hot but a solid when cooled. You know what that means? This kind of food contains fat, fat, and more fat! Would you like that clogging up your arteries?

Another grossing out tactic is to look at the ingredients, calories and fat that are in foods of interest. Many fast food chains post such information on their websites. In Eric Schlosser's book, *Fast Food Nation*, he lists several ingredients of a certain fast food restaurant's shake. It is enough to make it less appetizing. The nutritional information can collectively turn you off to such unhealthy foods.

I think it is better to have a good mindset about the greasy, unhealthy food. We do convince ourselves of many things. Some are convinced that they are the best person in the office, or the ugliest person in the world. We make rules about what is acceptable and unacceptable. If we can convince ourselves of such factors, why can't we convince ourselves that certain foods are too gross for us? It seems like a simple thing to do. Focus on something that is both very unhealthy and very tempting to eat. Try to convince yourself about something awful that is associated with it. Sometimes undesirable or unhealthy ingredients can help gross you out. Research some of these ingredients, and I am sure you will find enough information to turn you off. A big ingredient that gets negative attention is corn syrup and palm oil. Do what you can to turn yourself off to foods that are bad for you.

CHAPTER 34

The Supermarket Frenzy

The supermarket could be detrimental to our health. Some are not affected by this house of food, but the old me sure was. I know there are many of you out there just like me who have had struggles with weight. Supermarket visits put added stresses on our will to eat right. The food choices are endless, from the very healthy to the extremely unhealthy. And guess which group yours truly used to frequent? Of course, the answer is the unhealthy food groups. Supermarket shopping became very challenging for me. If it wasn't enough that I had purchased fattening foods to pig out on at home, I made sure I had some right by my side while driving home from the supermarket so starvation would not occur during the short trip home! It was doubly bad when there were free food samples. Some days had people in plain view with portable electric burners, cooking a greasefest of foods. If cooked samples were not available, then the fattening cheese spreads, dressings, candy, dips, and chips were present in abundance. Those little samples of chocolate covered somethings, fried somethings, and cakes lead to eating more food than I should have had in one meal! From the food I purchased to the free food on display, I was doomed.

The old me used to eat a small meal before food shopping. Eating before shopping is what I learned from countless shows and articles. Regardless, I made room for the free samples. One supermarket in particular had lots and lots of samples. There were stations all around the store, and I just had to try as many foods as possible. The food samples were rarely healthy and I would make many trips to ingest the grease and the grime! Therefore, having a small meal before food shopping was pointless. True food addicts will make room for what is offered in a supermarket. It is tough to turn down a free sample.

If I did not have enough free samples (which was usually the case), I would take one of my purchased items and eat it in the car. In fact, regardless of the number of free samples available, I would always find an excuse to eat newly purchased food while driving. I could finish at least a half a bag of potato chips while driving from the store to home. Sometimes I would eat nuts that I purchased or even chocolates. My desire for food was great and I just had to have something to tide me over on the short journey home. Looking back, I saw this was sad and desperate.

I had to make dramatic changes in the way I shopped for food. First of all, I made a list and stuck to it. The only exception was buying fruits and vegetables that were not on the list. For instance, corn was not on my list, but upon my arrival, I saw it was on sale and had to take advantage of the great price. Since it is healthy, it is worth purchasing, deviating from the list. I steer clear of samples. Most of the time others are flocking to the sample stands, which makes it easy to pass by. I would have to make an extra effort to shove myself in there and get some food. If there is some kind of opening, I try to walk quickly by and not even look at the free offerings.

There are two additional ways to avoid samples, the first of which is to gross yourself out. I go into more detail in the *Gross Yourself Out While You Are Out* chapter. Think of all the germy hands that delve into the free samples. Think of where these dirty hands have been. You will not be as tempted to dive into it yourself. The second way is to brush teeth just before going to the supermarket. It is less appetizing to eat something with a fresh, clean, minty mouth.

Some of us do not have time to cook and may occasionally grab items from the prepared foods section/counter. These selections are vast compared to when I was growing up. In my day, prepared foods meant cold cuts and various salads (e.g. potato salad, chicken salad, egg salad). Now selections include chicken parmesan, grilled salmon, chicken piccata, ribs, lasagna, beef sirloin tips, and crab cakes. There are soup choices galore, most of them in the creamy, more fattening category. Sides include mashed potatoes, carrots, potato pancakes, mixed vegetables, seasoned rice, and other wonderful additions. Prepared foods are great to have once in awhile, but should not be a daily staple in one's diet. Though an item looks healthy, it could be loaded with butter or oil, tremendously increasing the fat content. If I am in a time pinch and do need to rely on the prepared foods, I choose the grilled chicken. I never choose dishes that have some kind of sauce on them. Most likely it is a cream sauce and is of course very fattening. For me, I request the smallest piece of grilled chicken that they have. Usually that is four ounces (¼ pound), the ideal portion size for any meat or poultry dish I choose. For sides, I choose vegetables that look like they are not soaked in butter. The mashed potatoes at the one supermarket I frequent does not have a lot of butter, so I will have about a half a cup of that for my portion size. My family enjoys the grilled chicken as well, but I have no qualms about buying their favorite fatty entrees. After all, it is a sometime thing, not an all time thing. Therefore, I am satisfied with my selection and they are satisfied with theirs.

I also purchase ¼ pound of either chicken salad or tuna salad. This is a single portion for me. These salads have to look more "dry," which means less mayonnaise. Some chicken and tuna salads look like they are swimming in mayonnaise. If that is the case, I do not order them.

As mentioned before, I used to make sure all my favorite goodies were in the front seat with me so I could sample them on that car ride home. Of course this practice has changed. No, I do not just purchase fruits and vegetables. I do purchase chips and nuts for me and my family, but I make sure that all grocery bags are put in the trunk, away from me. Do not even try to put these items in the back seat. A food maven like me would make the extra effort to retrieve it. I would find a way, especially when waiting at a red light. The same could happen to you if you have such a strong craving. Paper products and other non tempting items can certainly be within reach, but put the tempting items in the trunk.

Taking proactive approaches such as these will make life easier, healthier, and less likely to lead to failure. The smaller steps taken can lead to even greater results.

CHAPTER 35

Take A Vacation, But Don't Take A Vacation From Exercise

People have great misconceptions about vacations. They feel enough calories will be burned sightseeing, swimming, and even lounging. I once read that an average person has to walk approximately 120 yards, the length of a football field, to burn off one plain M&M? Double that distance for one peanut M&M! Do an internet search as to how much exercise it will take to burn off a certain treat and you will be surprised. There is a lot of work involved in burning off goodies! So if it takes so much effort to burn off smaller intake, how long do you think it will take to burn off a creamed soup, lots of rolls, chicken parmesan, alcoholic beverages, and that nice piece of cake? Casual walking around will not burn off as much as you think.

Aside from portion control, exercising is needed to keep down the pounds. Do not fall into the trap by saying you went on vacation to relax, not to exercise. Touring and such is not laying around, relaxing. People mostly do more on vacation than what they do in their regular lives. So why not put exercise on your list of things to do? Even if lying around is the main part of the vacation, exercise is key.

Before I sought a healthier lifestyle, I made many unhealthy choices on vacation. Sure I made such poor choices in my everyday life, but on vacation it was worse. I tried to eat as much as I could on cruises. After all, I <u>had</u> to get my money's worth. If I passed by the burger joint near the pool that served unlimited burgers, fries, hot dogs, and tacos, I would grab a burger and fries. After all, it was free, part of my cruise cost. It also smelled great as I walked by. I made sure to attend all midnight buffets and afternoon teas. The ice cream machine was always on my route to somewhere, so I would have several cones of ice cream a day. If I could not decide on two desserts while in the dining room, I would have both. The server happily gave me what I wanted. On cruises, there is no etiquette to having seconds and thirds... On other vacations, I ordered huge meals for breakfast, lunch, and dinner. Appetizers were ordered for lunch and dinner, as well as large desserts. Meal selections were never healthy. Exercise was nonexistent. Though the ships we cruised on and the hotels we stayed at had lovely exercise areas filled with a plethora of machines, I never used any of them. I convinced myself that I would be exercising while sightseeing. I was completely out of control.

I made a mistake on a vacation during my healthy lifestyle change. We went on a seven night cruise. For those of you who are unfamiliar with this type of vacation, cruises equal lots of good food. Fortunately, my healthy lifestyle change prevented me from eating double desserts like I used to. And midnight buffets were no longer part of my itinerary. My plan was to take a break from exercise. My cruise was going to be filled with activities, enough to keep me busy and burn calories in the process. Boy, was I wrong! The cruise did have a great many activities but my food intake did not balance my amount of calories burned. I admit that I did overdo it a bit on the food. My eating did not consist of carrot sticks and celery! No way! The meals I chose did not come from the "heart smart" menu. I did eat, but what I didn't do was exercise. After all, I was on vacation. I wanted to relax and lounge around. Land excursions involved lots of walking, but not enough. I worked out once at the ship's fine spa. Other than that, I sat and played bingo, lounged around the pool, took a five minute walk on deck, played ping pong, and sat around, taking in the sights and shows. When I returned home, my weight gain was ten pounds! It took me a week to put it on and two months to take it off! It was a lousy price to pay. On the bright side, the weight gain was an "improvement," since I usually gained an average of fifteen pounds after a vacation.

When the next vacation came around, I did things differently. We spent a week in Cape May, NJ and got a room with a kitchenette. We brought our own food and had a lot of healthy options to choose from. We ate breakfast and lunches in the room. We would tour, but made sure we came back to the room for a meal or packed sandwiches in a cooler to have while we were on the move. Then out the door we would go! Dinner was always at a restaurant. I avoided all creamy soups, and stuck to a salad with a lighter dressing that was always ordered on the side. Appetizers were not ordered at all. My dinner was not fried, creamed, or sautéed. It was broiled steak or a shrimp dish. Vegetables always accompanied the main dish. I requested that nothing be cooked in butter, including the vegetables. Every evening I visited the hotel's gym. Quite honestly, it was far from a true gym. It was the size of our hotel room - nothing fancy. It had two treadmills and two elliptical machines; this was all I needed to burn off some calories. After my son went to bed, I worked out for a half hour to an hour. This really felt good, especially after eating a meal at a restaurant. After working out, I did not feel as weighed down. By the end of the vacation, I gained a mere two pounds. This weight gain was easily taken off in two days.

For my next Cape May trip, we selected a hotel that did not have exercise equipment at all. It was a little nicer than the previous hotel, so we made the change. However, I had to find a way to compensate for the gym loss. I could not think the old way and just substitute touring, casually walking around, as my exercise. Weeks before the trip, I scoped out gyms and found one that was about ten minutes from the hotel. I paid for a four day membership, which held me to a personal commitment. There was no way I would personally let a day go to waste, so there I was at the gym. I would go mainly in the evenings while my son was asleep and my husband was with him. The deciding factor for the gym was the closing time. I picked the gym that had the latest hours and was able to work out after the excitement of the day. For some, morning workouts are best, but evenings worked out for many reasons. Additionally, evening workouts helped when a meal did not sit well with me. It was nice to work out and feel better for it afterwards. The scale I brought with me helped me get myself to the gym. After eating out, I would return to the room and weigh myself. Not happy with the weight on the scale display, I practically "ran" to the gym!

The following year was another wonderful cruise. I know I had to change my strategies. It was the same cruise, the same good food. My strategy changed a lot. Aside from the fun activities from last year, a new one had to be added - the gym. This time, I visited the spa more often. I actually worked out, even if it was for 30 minutes. At least it was something. I sent Robert and Joseph to play ping pong or foosball while I worked out. There was no sense having them cooped up in their room, waiting for me. They got to have fun while I exercised. Of course my workouts were much more fun aboard ship. The treadmills and elliptical machines overlooked the magnificent ocean. What amazing views to see while exercising!

Did I gain some weight? Yes, but not as much! I am only human, and the food was good. I made the right choices, but had too much of it. For instance, I normally do not eat multi course meals. I may have a small salad, followed by my main course. Most often I just have a main course. This time I had an appetizer and the main course for both lunch and dinner. Fortunately, I made healthier choices. The good news is that it took me four days to take off what little I gained instead of the two months it took me from the prior year!

The key to gaining less on vacation is to have a game plan. If you are dining out in restaurants, use my advice to select "smarter" dishes. If it is unlimited eating such as on a cruise or an all inclusive resort, plan not to eat whenever food is seen. The way people eat on a cruise ship is horrifying! I would see people from our dinner seating go see the evening show right after their meals. This is great, but they would stop at the concession stand to purchase soft drinks, popcorn, and candy. Wait a minute? Didn't they just eat twenty minutes ago? People were crowding to get to the 11 pm dessert buffet, and piled on their plates as if they did not eat all day. The midnight buffet was packed! (Folks, I watched, and did not participate!) After a themed show that ended around 11 pm on the upper deck, people scrambled to get in line for the mini buffet. People piled on huge, greasy looking turkey legs, pizza, crepes, and tacos. Gee, that ought to sit well in their stomachs when they go to bed! What a weighed down, unhealthy feeling. I ought to know because the person I was long ago was one who raced to all of those special buffets. After all, I had to get my money's worth. In the meantime, I had to go to bed shortly after my feast, feeling overstuffed and a little sick.

Make sure you analyze the vacation before you go and make definitive plans. Without a solid game plan, your "eating behavior" wanders aimlessly, making huge mistakes along the way. Whatever the plan, be sure to work in exercise, whether it be for ten minutes, or more. Many hotels have gyms that will have just enough to do the job! Depending on your vacation destination, it is possible to find a gym that has "walk in" rates where a gym membership is not necessary. That could easily take care of the exercise part. Additionally, be sure to eat during the normal meal times. Avoid tea times (that usually involve breads, butter, and cakes), midnight buffets, and other extra "meals."

A great option worth executing before a non cruise vacation is to plan restaurants ahead of time and investigate the menus. Some people travel and randomly choose a place to eat at that moment. This could be detrimental to health! Some restaurants have terrible, unhealthy foods. After looking at some menus, I have deemed some restaurants to be fried food fests, to put it mildly. Meals are fried, sautéed, and fried! Gee, did I mention fried? Some items are baked, but are fattening. For instance, I saw <u>baked</u> mozzarella sticks. It may be baked, which is a healthier option, but is all that cheese concentrated in that dish really healthy? Yech!

When I plan a vacation, I always target restaurants for various days of our trip. I do a lot of surfing on the internet. I have found restaurants in theme parks that have broiled seafood platters. Surprisingly, I found a theme park restaurant that served tofu in a mango sauce. (Sorry, I know there are a lot of tofu haters out there. However, I love tofu and was glad to find this dish in a theme park eatery.) Theme parks are known for their fast food choices. Nowadays, healthier choices are incorporated into the menus. It is better to find these restaurants ahead of time. Vacations can be tiring, and will most likely lead you to give up and find the first restaurant you find. This establishment may or may not offer the best choices for you. Having a list with addresses/directions will make the chances of finding better food much greater. True this is one extra thing to put on a vast list of things to do, but we have to make the extra effort to look and feel great.

As situations occur, it is oftentimes difficult to plan ahead to find a restaurant. Sometimes we find ourselves in an area and will choose some eatery in the proximity of where we are. If that is the case, check out the menu before being seated. Many post their menus just outside of the restaurants. Take a gander and scope out what would be acceptable. If it is difficult to find a semi healthy meal, move on. If a menu is not posted, enter and ask the host or hostess to see a menu before being seated. Make your decision right then and there.

Wandering aimlessly, eating aimlessly, will not help reach goals. Believe me, we are all worth the extra efforts, so go that extra mile.

If you do gain weight after your return, do not give up. If you follow these vacation tips, you may still put on the pounds, but not as much as you normally would. When I gained a few pounds on the last vacation, I was not happy at all. However, I asked myself if I had a good time. I did, so it was worth it. And the increase in weight was not the fifteen pounds I would usually gain. Instead of throwing a pity party for myself, I decided to be happy. There were lots of things to be grateful for, so I maintained that positive spirit and was motivated to press forward, losing the extra weight. With that spirit, I dropped the dreaded pounds and was back to normal. If you are in a similar situation, dust yourself off and get right to work. Getting back on track will lead to weight loss success. But as you plan a vacation in general, food and exercise must be part of the planning as well.

The Dining Out
Chapter Series

CHAPTER 36

Don't Get Your Money's Worth

One of the many excuses for eating a lot is getting "the money's worth." This thought process is often applied to restaurants, vacations, and all inclusive types of meal plans. Some even apply it to a party of some sort. For instance, if a gift is given for a wedding, some have the mindset to eat a lot to get their money's worth for what they paid out. The latter did not appeal to me as much, but if I went to a buffet, I wanted to get my money's worth and eat as much as I could. If my workplace had a holiday luncheon, I had to make sure I ate the most expensive foods and lots of it. I stayed away from salads because that was the "cheap food." In my mind, the foods that were fried and swimming in cream sauces were higher in value, so it was much more important to eat the more expensive food. If I was at a restaurant, I also wanted to get my money's worth by clearing my plate and eating all the extras that were given me such as bread and salad bar food. If I was on a cruise, I definitely had to get my money's worth by eating as often as I could. Although I never ate at midnight in my everyday life, I would make sure to change my ways if a midnight buffet was on the itinerary. Additionally, I would never pass over a special dessert buffet. After all, I just had to get my money's worth! And of course I am not alone. Millions of people feel the same way.

People even want to get money's worth at someone else's expense! If you do not believe me, check out those who flock around the free food samples at the supermarket, fair, or expo. Some will even knock you down or cut the line, just to get some of that fattening sample. One was even willing to knock over my then seven year old son for a piece of burger. Food is a big deal to some. These individuals thrive on getting things for free, so they might as well have lots of that free stuff, knocking out anyone or anything that gets in the way!

Do people actually get their money's worth? Not really. People end up with a stuffed feeling, more damage to their bodies, and many gained pounds. There is no true satisfaction after eating everything we could. If people try to get their money's worth more often, health problems arise, actually costing individuals more, regardless if there is medical insurance. Gaining weight does not help people get their money's worth. When I gained fifteen pounds after a cruise, was it really worth it to eat every chance I could? Was the overstuffed feeling worth it, where I felt so bad that I did not feel like participating in the amazing activities that were planned? Was I really getting my money's worth?

To sum it up for this chapter, do not have that *I have to get my money's worth* mentality. Eat regular meals on vacation, regardless if the foods are unlimited. As highlighted in the Supermarket Frenzy chapter, bypass those free samples. Keep in mind those germy customers who come in contact with the samples, and just focus on your shopping. If visiting a buffet, limit it to one buffet trip for the main meal, including salad and the entrée. Fill one plate flat, not mountainous. Use a small plate for a dessert. Do not be tempted to visit again and again to get the most out of your money.

We need to drop this "getting the most for our money" mentality when it comes to food. Stuffing our faces, gaining weight, and feeling lousy are not ways of getting our money's worth. It just makes us feel more worth - less.

CHAPTER 37

The Main Meal at the Restaurant

One of the most difficult things to do is to order a main meal. Sure it is easy to pick an entrée that is creamy, fatty, and so on. It is more difficult to choose something sensible. For me, seeing Chicken Française, Beef Burgundy, chicken parmesan, fried shrimp, and other "niceties" on the menu would get me hooked, steering me away from my plans to choose sensibly.

Planning ahead is key. Most people know in advance that they are going to a restaurant for lunch or dinner. Sure things can be sporadic and done on a whim, but most people do make lunch or dinner plans. If you know you are going to dine out, take it easy on the meals prior to or following the big restaurant visit. If dinner is the dining out meal for example, go easy on the breakfast and lunch, eating less than you normally would. This allows you to splurge on the meal...to a point.

Before even choosing a restaurant, make sure there are items on the menu that you can eat. For instance, if the place has only fried foods, do not even eat there. Obviously choices will not be healthy ones. Nowadays menus can easily be viewed on the internet so you know dining fare ahead of time. Entrees should consist of grilled or broiled foods. Good salad options are important too. Of course a good dessert selection is important! Yes, dessert is important to those who crave the sweet stuff. It is important to have the right dessert and feel satisfied. If the old me hated my dessert that I had at a restaurant, I would return home and immediately make up for it. Ice cream, cookies, and chocolates were my "friends." Therefore, choose the restaurant wisely for better choices and more satisfaction.

Let us take it one step at a time. First, stay clear from appetizers and soups. Stick to the main entrée and dessert. You are allowed to live it up, to a point! Refraining from appetizers could be a challenge. What used to weaken me, making it difficult to avoid appetizers, is when the server would ask, "Would you like to start off with an appetizer? We have mozzarella sticks, wings, nachos, sliders...." I hated that. If only they would simply ask if we wanted an appetizer. Mentioning some of the choices made it very difficult to avoid, especially because I was, and still am, a food lover. Restaurants are counting on that, hoping to rake in more money by tempting diners with some of the delectable, mostly unhealthy choices. And of course servers like it when patrons order more items because the greater the bill, the greater the tip.

The old me used to cave in and order the first thing mentioned that appealed to me. Now I tune out what the server says. All I hear is "blah, blah, blah," and let he or she talk without paying attention to the words. When there is a pause, I say, "No thank you," and give my order. Another trick is to interrupt. Here is my typical scenario.

SERVER: Would you like to start off with an appetizer? We have wing-

LORI: Uh, no thank you - sorry to interrupt. I'll just have the...

In the midst of this, I sometimes vary the conversation with mentioning that I need to make room for dessert. I do have dessert just about every time I dine out, and you will find out what I do in the next chapter which is dedicated to just desserts.

When placing an order, do not be afraid to ask a server how

the food is prepared. Is it broiled in butter? Does it have a cream or butter sauce? Is it fried? Can you have the sauce on the side or is the dish prepared with the sauce already in it? Find out and make minor changes. For instance, ask for that sauce on the side. Request that the entrée be broiled without butter. Finding out how food is prepared and fine tuning can really help.

Certain meals come with a choice of size. For instance, some salads are either half or full portion. Some steaks on the menu come in four ounce, eight ounce, and even a whopping pounder. Burgers could also be various sizes. Regardless of these choices, always go for the smallest size. You will not starve, trust me! It will be satisfying. Whether I have the smallest burger or steak, I have never left a restaurant starving or even a bit hungry. Sometimes, as the saying goes, our eyes are bigger than our stomachs. My husband, who is used to ordering medium portions, now orders the smallest sizes of food. He says he does not miss the few extra ounces less of food and his waistline does not miss it either!

While you are waiting for your main meal, you are not out of the woods. See all the road blocks we are faced with just for dining out? The appetizer culprits are away, but what about the bread? The server usually follows up with a lovely bread basket. Some have big, fluffy rolls and crisp, crusty breads. Don't forget the small packages of butter that are enough for three times the number of people at the table. When the three of us go out, I sometimes find enough butter where when dividing it up, we can each have three to four small packages/pads! Now that is a lot of butter! If it is not butter that is presented, then it is the small swimming pool of oil that is set on the table. It is a generous, vast bowl of olive oil that has a few herbs swimming in it. It is a sea of cholesterol clogging liquid!

There are two smart choices you can make when it comes to bread. You can ask for a bread basket, but for the number of rolls that corresponds to the number of people in your group who will have bread. In my family, all three of us eat bread, so I will ask for a basket of only three rolls. If you do have bread, and the restaurant serves that swimming pool of oil, request it not be brought to the table at all. I ask for butter instead, which they do have. Use the butter sparingly, just for flavor. It is a healthier option than dunking it in that swimming pool of fat. Secondly, you can kindly ask to not have bread brought to the table. A lot of our main meal choices are starchy. For lunch items, sometimes sandwiches are the main meal, so bread is a big part of what we are eating anyway. Therefore, bread is not a necessity. Besides, it is something we eat while we are "bored," waiting for our food to come. We will not starve without it and will be satisfied when our meals arrive. So perhaps for some, not having bread at all is best.

However, let's say that bread is on the table or we have that urge to grab something. After all, we are waiting for the food and are bored. Instead of waiting and craving, keep busy. I bring my iPod and play a game with my family. I do not just sit there and ignore them. There are also games on people's cell phones. We play a game that everyone can participate in. For instance, we play a word game and everyone calls out words to add to the list. We try to increase our points for every game that we play. Sometimes I take scrap paper out of my purse and write a long word down, such as the word "information." We try to find as many words as we can that are three letters or more. Sometimes we play Hangman either on paper or on the iPod. Playing simple games such as these takes away from the doldrums of waiting for food to arrive. I make sure it is something we can all be a part of. There are too many scenarios of individuals utilizing electronic devices, ignoring all at the table. When we dine out, we communicate and interact. Therefore, use that family time to choose short activities all can participate in before the food arrives.

My entrée selections vary, depending on the restaurant and my mood. I try to avoid the fried dishes or high fat meats such as duck. If I want something a little higher in calories and fat, I will exercise in the morning a little extra to compensate. Additionally, if it is a dinner, I will have a smaller lunch or vise versa if I am dining out for lunch. Here are some of my typical restaurant choices:

- Salad with grilled chicken or shrimp. Dressing is always ordered on the side. I then put an equivalent of two tablespoons of dressing on the salad and mix. Another trick is to ask for two tablespoons of dressing. Dip your fork in the dressing, and then into your salad. You still get the flavor of the salad dressing, which for once is not drowning the food. Avoid salads that have a lot of fattening ingredients such as nuts. If it does, ask for the nuts on the side and have a tablespoon of those. Of course, avoid salads all together that have fattening main ingredients such as chicken fingers and cheese. Although cheese does not seem like a main ingredient it could be. Some restaurants generously put a lot of cheese all over the salad. More about salads in the *Salad Sense* chapter.

- Shrimp skewers over rice. Shrimp is so low in calories and fat. Fried shrimp obviously is not, but grilled shrimp is ideal. Ask to hold the butter and oil. Sometimes the shrimp is cooked with oil.

- Chicken or shrimp fajitas - request that the skillet has zero to little oil. Perhaps take it further and request it be prepared with nonstick cooking spray. Four tortillas are usually small. Restaurants have really cut back nowadays. Use two tablespoons of cheese. Avoid the guacamole - ask the server not to include it in your meal to avoid temptation. Sour cream is oftentimes served, so limit that to a tablespoon. Salsa and vegetables can be enjoyed in unlimited quantities. Request that the food not be cooked in oil, but just the seasonings alone. This will help reduce a great amount of fat.

- 4 to 6 ounce steak and baked potato. Many steakhouses list the weight of the steaks, such as for filet mignons. Go for the smallest portion offered and ask that the steak not be flavored with butter. Sometimes steaks are prepared as such to make them moist. Do not request butter or sour cream to be put directly on the baked potato. Ask for sour cream on the side, or else it will be loaded up on the potato. Sour cream will be tasty enough where you will not miss the butter. If sour cream is not to your liking, use butter sparingly. I try to avoid butter and will use sour cream, parmesan cheese, or salsa for flavoring.

- Grilled Salmon or flounder - make sure you request that the fish not be cooked in butter, but a nonstick spray instead.

- Steamed or grilled crab legs! Yum! There is a place I love that serves crabs. They always put the butter on the side (which I do not use). The process of opening the crab legs slows down my eating and I receive the message that I am full before eating a lot of food.

These are some suggestions to get you on the right track. These choices are reasonable, and will not put on the calories and fat that some of my old favorites used to do!

Now that the entrée selection is taken care of, you have to consider the sides. The potato (with toppings on the side to use sparingly) has been discussed. Sometimes there are other choices besides the baked potato such as fries, mixed vegetables, applesauce, coleslaw, or a featured vegetable. Any vegetable ordered, whether mixed or featured should have a special request - no butter. So often I have received vegetables that are greasy and have pools of yellow, melted butter, underneath them. This adds so many calories and especially fat. Coleslaw, depending how it is made, can be fattening as well. Fries of course are often greasy, so that would not be my side of choice. Go for the applesauce or some kind of vegetable without butter.

The next thing to be concerned about are the portions that are served to you. Some restaurants have cut back, and have been serving paltry amounts of food. Others are in the "mega amount" zone, piling plates high with food. Regardless of the amount served, portions must be adjusted. I am going to show you how to get the right portion.

First of all, ask for a take - home container as soon as you receive your meal. It will be right at your side and you will be more out to packing up the meal. Sometimes waiting for a server to bring a container will force you to eat more in the meantime. Some restaurants like to have servers take unfinished portions in the back and pack it up. Most will appreciate your request, for it is one less thing the server has to do. It is for your own good for another reason. Sometimes accidents happen, and food ends up on a dirty counter or even on the floor when trying to quickly transfer leftovers to a container. I once saw a server drop a container in a rush. Some of the food oozed out onto the floor. She quickly scooped it up and continued on her way to deliver it to the customer! Gross! That is why I pack my own leftovers. Doing this makes it more sanitary and it alleviates work for the servers. If the take - home container is often tempting for journeys home, put it in the trunk so you will not pick at it. Just remember to take it out of the trunk and put the contents in the refrigerator once you get home!

A good meat/poultry/fish portion is usually the size of a deck of cards. A good idea is to take a card and study the size. This is roughly 3 ½ inches long and 2 ¼ inches wide. Even practice drawing it and measure to see if you got the size down in your mind. Another option is to bring an old card with you. It is portable and can fit into any wallet. There is another good trick for measuring in the *For Good Measure* chapter where it describes weighing a controlled portion of meat/poultry/fish at home and use an item (e.g. wallet, compact mirror) that you would have on you if in a restaurant. Use this item to compare sizes. This helps in size approximation and can give you a better sense of portion control. If the entrée is a big piece of chicken or steak, cut it to that size and immediately put the excess in the take-out container. If the entrée is smaller pieces of food such as shrimp, or chicken from fajitas, aggregate them together to form that shape. Then place any excess in the take-out container. Be sure not to fool yourself. Some people will collect the food into that shape, but will make it a mountain! Be sure the thickness is about a half an inch thick, not more that ¾ of an inch.

Sizes of sides also has to be taken into consideration. Portion sizes need not apply to non starchy vegetables without butter, so enjoy! Usually a side of applesauce is small, so the portion size is not a major concern. Starchy vegetables should comprise of a cups worth. To visualize this, keep portion sizes of starchy vegetables such as corn or potatoes to the size of a tennis ball.

More and more restaurants offer a 500 calorie or less selection. I have tried many of these dishes at various restaurants and have never been dissatisfied. This type of selection can make entrée selection a lot easier. Portion size is no longer a concern.

Please do not be overly consumed with sizes. This is not rocket science - things do not have to be precise to the 0.01 milligram. This is a guideline to control portions and to prevent us from eating whatever is on our plates, which is usually too much for one person to consume in one sitting.

I measure my food at home, which makes it easier over time for dining out. Because I got into the practice of measuring, I am able to eyeball something and know its size. Regardless, when dining out, I use my compact mirror to measure the main entrée portion size. It is the perfect size for a four ounce piece of steak or chicken, for instance, and makes for a good guide. Such guides are important, or else a tablespoon could turn into a half a cup portion and that deck of cards shape will turn into three decks! And remember that eyeballing should be used only for dining out. If we have the ability to grab a measuring utensil such as in the house, let's do it and not resort to approximations.

Another option to self selection of the main course and sides is sharing entrees. This is not what most would assume. I would personally be embarrassed to order a meal for one because that would make me look cheap. This is a different kind of sharing. First of all, you need a willing eating partner, whether it is a love, friend, or relative. One can order a healthy salad entree with dressing on the side. Another can order a meal of chicken, fish, or beef that is at least a little on the healthy side and that both parties wish to eat. Both entrees can be split and shared with one another so each person could have a half a salad and a half a main entrée. This greatly reduces the calorie and fat intake. Each can enjoy a little healthy, a little semi-healthy meal.

Whatever you eat, take it slow! Do not quickly devour your food. Remember the *Stop the Shoveling and the Stuffing* chapter? Ask for a shrimp fork and/or tea spoon, depending on what you are eating. These small utensils will help slow down your eating. You will also get to enjoy the food longer, not feeling deprived. Break the food into smaller pieces. For instance, I will cut an individual scallop or piece of shrimp into three pieces. If the entrée is pieces as meat, as seen in sirloin tips, cut each piece into three. Most people will pop them whole; some may even stuff a few in at a time. To slow the eating down and also get maximum enjoyment of the taste, cut the food up into smaller pieces.

If at all possible, dining out should be considered a treat, and should not be a part of everyday eating. I personally dine out once a week. On a rare occasion, it could be twice a week. The other days should consist of packing meals on the go or eating sensibly at home.

Now read on to learn how to handle dessert, the "sweetest" part of the meal!

CHAPTER 38

When It Comes to Dessert – Be a Kid or Split!

Desserts are so important to so many. It is not dinner without a sweet treat, especially when a particular restaurant is famous for its desserts. How in the world can we resist them?

I must say that I rarely pass up on the dessert. The only exception is when I dine with friends. Most turn down dessert, which makes it easy for me to jump on the bandwagon and do the same. I won't sit with a dessert while everyone else stares. When I am with my family, it is a whole other ballgame.

I want to enjoy dessert and I realize I do not need a lot to feel satisfied. Therefore, I have a choice. I could either order a kid's size dessert or I could have half of a regular dessert. If we visit an ice cream parlor, I order either a kid's cup or kid's cone. No one has ever denied me yet. No one says that I cannot order it because I am not a child. There were times I went for dessert with friends, and never was I denied that smaller size. It has just enough ice cream for that amazing taste. The old me would look at the size of the cups and would convince myself that smaller sizes were not enough for me and would not be satisfying. One of my old friends felt the same way and ordered a pint! In reality, the smaller size is just as satisfying as the larger size. The first few bites are heavenly, but soon after the dessert becomes dull and not as flavorful. Your taste buds get used to the flavor and subsequent tastes are not as enjoyable as the first few. The difference of having a smaller size is that you won't be overstuffed and even sick like you would if you had the mega size. And of course, you will be putting fewer calories and less fat into your system!

I often enlist my husband's help to share dessert with me. We choose a dessert we both enjoy and I ask the server to split it. My husband remarked on several occasions that he was satisfied with half a slice just as much as a whole slice. I couldn't agree more. The first bite is the most heavenly. The second bite is good. The third bite is okay. It gets to a point where it doesn't have that initial great taste that bursts with flavor. From that point on, you end up putting extra calories and fat into you without really tasting it.

Sometimes my husband gets a little greedy; he wants his own dessert. In that case, we then get our own dessert. I will ask the server to split my dessert, but to pack the other half to take home. Most of the time, however, my husband is very willing to share.

Therefore, split your desserts. You can even save money, which is an added bonus! Nowadays desserts in restaurants cost around eight or nine dollars. One less dessert saves that much and over months, can save amounts that are far significant. Not only does half a dessert help your health, but your wallet as well! A thinner waist could mean a fatter wallet! Who can ask for anything more? And of course, life will be sweeter for your taste and your waist!

CHAPTER 39

Another Time to be a Kid

Once we get older, there is little time to be a kid. Now there is a chance - get a kid's meal. Of course no restaurant in its "right mind" would allow an adult to order a children's meal. What restaurants cannot do is deny such an order for takeout. What can they do or say? If you are picking up meals for your family, is the restaurant owner going to ask for proof of the children who are going to eat these meals? If so, find another restaurant! Most of the time you can pick up a takeout order and simply pay and go without interrogation. Go for the children's meals; for the most part, these kiddie portions are just the right size. You can still enjoy normal food without having a huge portion to deal with.

One time I really had a craving for a sub sandwich, or hoagie as some of you call it. My choices were either a seven inch or fourteen inch sandwich. Neither was an option because the serving sizes were too large. I could not split a seven inch sandwich at the time because I was far from home and did not have an insulated lunch bag with me. I was about to give up on the idea until my eyes focused on something wonderful - a kid's box lunch. This was exactly what I needed. It came with a four inch sandwich, which was perfect. It also includes carrot sticks, a choice of water or a boxed juice, and animal crackers. The portion size was ideal, and was able to enjoy a sandwich that was just the right size.

As an aside, it is important to be mindful of choices when deciding what goes into a sub sandwich. Avoid the oils, mayonnaise, bacon, and such. For instance, the sandwich I have at times is roast beef with provolone cheese. I request a small amount of honey mustard, and then have lettuce, tomatoes, and onions. I get a lot of taste for less fat and calories.

Restaurants, including the chain eateries, have a nice selection of kid entrees. They are not all burgers, macaroni and cheese, or chicken fingers. Many selections include a small pizza (usually equivalent to 1 ¼ slices of regular pizza, not too shabby), grilled chicken, small burger sliders, chicken quesadillas, and spaghetti and meat balls. Again, portions are usually smaller and are just the right size.

Restaurants, sub shops, pizza parlors, and the like are starting to enhance food choices for children, including healthier choices. Some even incorporate apple slices as a side. Why not take advantage of these offerings? You can enjoy favorite foods without stuffing yourself. Another added bonus is that these meals are much cheaper. Once again, you save big and gain little!

CHAPTER 40

Pizza Palooza!

The reality is that we do not always eat high quality food from restaurants. We do not always achieve that sit down dinner. Pizza is one of the fast foods many of us often seek. How wonderful to phone ahead and have it delivered right to your door in the midst of the rushing around and work! It is also easy to call ahead and pick up a pizza while on the go. The pizzeria gives you paper plates and such and voila! You have an instant meal. Some diets will recommend staying away from foods like pizza. I say we are only human, and most of us do crave this incredible food from time to time. That is why I could never follow a diet that required giving up carbohydrates such as pizza. I cannot live without pizza forever and do enjoy a slice from time to time. Pizza is a common favorite food, so completely eliminating it, never to be eaten again is unrealistic. Such eliminations also lead to "falling off the healthy eating wagon" and going back to old bad eating habits.

There are many options I have for working pizza into meals from time to time. I do make a one slice rule. I made a rule for myself that I can have pizza no more than twice a month and no more than one slice in one sitting. For some, the one slice rule may seem preposterous. Nonetheless, you are reading a book by someone who would eat five slices in one sitting! I must admit that

I did not instantaneously reduce my intake from five slices to one. As previously mentioned, I took it one slice at a time. Instead of five slices, I went for months with four slices. I then reduced it to three, and eventually got it down to one. If I was able to cut back on the pizza, so can you! If you ate many slices as I did, gradually reduce the number of slices eaten in one meal.

Once I get my slice of pizza to eat, I blot the top with a paper towel or napkin. This absorbs the oil from the hot cheese. After blotting the pizza, the paper towel is filled with oil/grease. It is better that it is on the paper towel than on your hips! If need be, use another paper towel once the first one gets saturated. This practice really does reduce the amount of fat that enters your system.

Another thing you can do is remove the cheese, cutting off a piece parallel to the crust, about an inch of cheese in depth. Take the cheese that was removed and give it to a friend or relative. If need be, donate it to the garbage! If placed on the side of the plate, it may become too tempting and will be eaten anyway. This of course defeats the purpose. Getting rid of it immediately is best. It does save on a few calories and a few grams of fat, so it is well worth it. Not immediately disposing the removed portion will most likely lead to failure. One of my friends who was dieting at the time would try something like this. She would eat half a cookie. When I first saw her do this, I had great admiration for her. I thought she had amazing control. Soon after, she ate the other half, therefore making the effort pointless. Getting rid of the other half immediately, either by giving it to someone else or putting it out of sight would be best and would lead to more success. So take that cheese off and hide it one way or another!

If you have the choice, order the Margarita (or sometimes spelled "Margherita, Margharita, et cetera…) pizza. A regular slice is loaded with cheese. The Margarita pizza has thin slices of fresh mozzarella cheese sporadically placed on the pizza. Therefore, less cheese, less fat. This kind of pizza is lightly smattered with cheese and sauce. It is less fattening than a regular slice. Encourage your family to get this kind of pizza. When I go out for pizza with friends, and I see the variety of slices to choose from, I go for the Margarita pizza. Try to avoid fattening toppings such as sausage, pepperoni, ham, cheese steaks (i.e. cheese steak pizza), and tortellini. Try to go for a regular slice of pizza without the toppings. Avoid deep dish pan pizzas. They tend to be very greasy and obviously have a lot more calories and fat. Have a side salad with a small amount of dressing if you think you will be starving with one slice of pizza. The salad will help you feel more fulfilled, but watch the fattening dressing! See the Salad Sense Chapter for more tips on having a healthier salad.

If you are at a friend's/relative's home, and pizzas are ordered for a group, kindly ask if the pizzeria sells slices. If so, ask if they have Margarita pizza and kindly request a slice. Also, most importantly, pay for the slice! It is a specialty pizza, and costs a little more. It would be an added cost to the host or hostess who could easily avoid the expense by ordering bulk plain pizzas. So be considerate and throw a five dollar bill in his or her direction! (The pizza slice does not cost that much, but it is a generous gesture!) Another option is to have the regular slice, but remove an inch of cheese from the crust.

Do not let anyone sucker you into having another slice. I always get people urging me to take the last slice or to not care about my eating plan for just this one day. As the saying goes, "Just say no." With practice and overall effort, you will find that you really do not need that extra slice of pizza. It does not make you enjoy the meal any better. Try to stay out of the room where the pizzas are. If they are out of your sight, the thoughts of having another slice will most likely be out of your mind!

Another option is to make your own pizza. I have an awesome

alternative that drastically cuts back on the calories and fat. Use a medium to large tortilla and add your sauce, cheese (I recommend three tablespoons of shredded mozzarella) and vegetable toppings. Bake at 350° for about ten to fifteen minutes and you have yourself a thin crust, crispy pizza. You can be creative with the tortillas because of the variety (e.g. pesto, tomato, whole wheat spinach tortillas). It is just as enjoyable! It looks large too, so it is visually satisfying. Feel free to top it with a lot of the unlimited vegetables such as onion, eggplant, broccoli, and spinach. Therefore, it will be satisfying to the eyes as well as to the stomach. Another option is to make a pizza on a pita or naan bread. Give it a shot!

Making subtle changes like the ones outlined in this chapter will allow you to easily incorporate it into your life without the higher cholesterol, fat, and weight gain! You do not have to deprive yourself and eliminate pizza for good. You can have your pizza slice and still be on the healthy eating track!

CHAPTER 41

Burger Blues

This chapter is about more than the standard beef burger. It includes veggie burgers, turkey burgers, and the like. Burgers of all sorts can really increase calories and fat intake. The burger alone could be fattening. The fat content could be high and may be mixed with other things to make it even more fattening such as cheese or bacon. In many restaurants, the burger is made on the same grill that greasy bacon, sausage, cheese steaks, and other greasy foods are cooked on. The bun it is on is usually thick and large, packing on too many calories, fat, and carbohydrates overall. Some establishments even butter the bun or roll! Then to add more calories and fat are the dreaded toppings. The lettuce, tomatoes, onions, and pickles are harmless. The cheese, mayonnaise, bacon, onion rings, ranch dressing, and such contribute a lot of calories and fat. Let's not forget the traditional greasy fries, the popular accompaniment. Collectively, the burger entrée is a concoction of calories and fat that will easily help pack on the pounds.

Unlike other diet/healthy eating books, I am not going to tell you to never eat this kind of food again. Depriving oneself of a good burger is unfair and can lead to breakdown of the healthy eating journey. What you can do is greatly reduce the calories and fat of a burger that is either made at home or enjoyed at a restaurant.

Let us start with the burger of choice. Of course it is tough to choose the quality of ground beef, but opt for lean beef if you can, especially when making it at home. Try not to get cheese or bacon mixed into the ground beef. Most of the time it is difficult to taste these additives in the burger, so omit these needless calories and fat. Speaking of fat, make sure you blot the burger with a napkin before eating or just after cooking. If there are toppings that are already on the burger, blot the bottom. It is so worth it and that blotted oil will not end up in your system.

If you are making a burger at home, do not use oil to coat the pan. Use a nonstick spray. The fat from the burger will also contribute to the nonstick effect, so nonstick spray is best. Oil has a lot of fat and truthfully, there is enough fat in the burger. Oil, therefore, is unnecessary.

In regards to the hamburger roll, have an open faced burger! Have the one half of the roll on the bottom and pile on healthy toppings (read on!). If you put the bread on top of the burger, you will not even notice that the bottom bread is missing. Only eat one part of the roll, either the top or bottom half. It is your choice, so go for either one. You really will not miss the two pieces of bread. You can still eat it with your hands. If you wish, put a piece of lettuce underneath to hold it in place better. As mentioned previously, I eat with a shrimp fork. I do eat sandwiches with a shrimp fork to slow down my eating. Burgers are one of the foods I eat with a fork and knife, so eating this open faced burger sandwich is easy for me and even helps me miss the bottom part of the bun even less.

Another low calorie, low fat option for a burger roll is a taco shell! I microwave the taco shell for fifteen seconds and place the burger in the shell. I stuff it with lettuce, tomatoes, and onions. I also drizzle a low fat dressing on it - no more than one tablespoon. One I like in particular is a peanut dressing. Voila! You have a taco burger. It is delicious. You get that crunch that is very satisfying.

If you want to change things up even more and stray from the traditional hamburger bun, try a small pita bread or even a soft flour tortilla. Most have a lot less calories and fat compared to a standard hamburger bun. This pita bread pocket allows for stuffing of your favorite ingredients. It is a great alternative and the burger still tastes great. The tortilla can also hold favorite ingredients, but it would be best to half the burger, placing the halves on top of each other. By doing this allows for more (healthy) ingredients to be added (e.g. lettuce, tomatoes, salsa, onions). There are so many varieties of pita bread and tortillas, so it will give a lot of variety each time if you venture.

Another way to enjoy a burger is to cook the tortilla! First, place the cooked burger in the center of a round tortilla. Place one slice of cheese on the burger and fold up the "edges" of the tortilla. Cook the burger/tortilla in a skillet, three minutes on each side. First cook with the folded (not smooth) side down to seal the burger in. The tortilla becomes crisp and makes for a very enjoyable meal.

Toppings have to be planned for as well. They quickly add up in calories and fat. One slice of cheese is plenty. If ordering out, request one slice of cheese. Two or more slices appear to be ideal, but that kind of desired quantity is all in the mind. One slice will taste just as good and you will not miss the extra slices of cheese. Load up the toppings with vegetables such as lettuce, tomatoes and onions, but avoid fattening foes like mayonnaise, bacon, and creamy dressings. A healthier option to creamy toppings is mixing one tablespoon of ketchup and one tablespoon of mustard. Put that on a burger for a great taste. It is a great substitute for creamy dressings, or even cheese. As previously mentioned, I will put a low calorie dressing on the burger instead of cheese. The dressing contributes a lot of flavor, and cheese is therefore not necessary or missed.

Another option when it comes to toppings is to ask for them on the side when ordering out. When you get the burger, you can blot the grease with a napkin and then add the toppings yourself. This may seem like an insignificant step, but what ends up on your napkin will not end up on your body!

Fries are fattening foes at eateries. Most often they are served as a side automatically. You do not have to settle for the traditional side of massive fries. Many restaurants offer substitutes at no extra charge. Either order vegetables, apple sauce, or coleslaw. One restaurant I frequent will substitute nacho chips and salsa. The chips are not massive, and it definitely contains fewer calories and fat compared to the fries. If substitutions are not listed on the menu, just ask. Most of the time I am surprised with the numerous healthy choices that I have. If you really want to enjoy the fries, tell the server that you want only twelve fries on your plate if they are the "shoestring" fries most often seen in fast food restaurants. If they are steak fries, the fatter ones, request only five. If I am dining out and if either my son or husband has fries on the side, I will pick off twelve shoestring fries or five steak fries. Most places give a copious amount of fries, so a family member is not deprived if someone else takes a few.

If you are cooking at home, make baked fries as opposed to the fryer/oil kind. There are frozen brands that can easily be baked in the oven instead of frying them. To make them more crisp, broil them during the last three minutes of cooking time. You can always slice potatoes thin, dip them in egg whites, sprinkle a seasoning on them such as Old Bay, and then bake at 350° for one hour. These are very satisfying, and you will not miss the grease!

Keep in mind that burgers should not be eaten every day. It should be a sometime meal. I know people who eat burgers everyday or a few times a week. Their reasoning is that it is convenient and they do not have time to eat something different. For those who internalized the "Drop The Excuses" chapter, you know the excuse is not valid. Excuses lead to failure, so to avoid that, drop the excuses and find healthy alternatives to replace that burger.

When looking at the big picture, you will see that the changes are subtle and can make significant differences. You end up getting to enjoy a food that you love without unnecessary calories and fat that will clog your arteries and your life!

CHAPTER 42

Salad Sense

There is a scenario that is very common in people's eating habits. A salad is ordered in an eatery "as is," with the consumer making no requests for modifications. That is, nothing is cut back, eliminated or changed. The person eats every bit of it, and then acts shocked about the weight gain the following day.

I used to play the victim when it came to food and weight loss. I could eat a salad the night before, gain weight the next day, and begin my dramatic rant as the victim of an unfair scam:

Why me? I was so good! I had a nice, healthy salad and I gained weight. The weight gain is not my fault. I don't understand!

The problem was that I was neither realistic nor truthful with myself. We can all lie and even fool ourselves. Let us analyze this "nice, healthy" salad further. Most of these meals include lettuce as the base. That should not contribute to weight gain. Vegetables such as broccoli, onions, tomatoes, cucumbers, and mushrooms can be included. So far so good, right? These are ingredients that have no fat and most diet plans allow for them in unlimited quantities. Now add bacon, chicken fingers, steak, two heaping ladles of dressing, cheeses, walnuts, pistachios, cashews, sunflower seeds, almonds, fried onions, olives, beans marinated in oil, croutons, Chinese noodles, and other fattening ingredients. This is when the salad goes sour - health wise, that is. The salad was nice in taste, but not healthy. If I really, really looked at those salads of the past, I would see that there were a great many fattening ingredients included. But let us take note that those aforementioned items help put on the pounds. Let us also keep in mind that in a super - sized portion world, these ingredients are put in salads in massive quantities. Unfortunately eateries are all about large portions so the said ingredients are greatly present Obviously that leads to more calories and fat than we need.

I order salads from restaurants all of the time, but I order smart. Dressings must be on the side. I will take two tablespoons of it for my salad. If I cannot measure it accurately and am in a restaurant, I will take three spoons of dressing and put it on my salad. If the dressing is thick, I will lightly dilute it with water to get more spreadability so it will spread through the salad better instead of remaining in a clump. If at a restaurant, ask the server for a small dish or cup to dilute the dressing. I sometimes refrain from adding dressing to my salad. Instead, I dip my fork in the dressing, then take a stab at the salad. Another option I choose from time to time is spreading the salad out on a flat plate. Try this! Ask for a dish instead of a bowl. If making a salad at home, spread the salad out in a rectangular container. The bowl allows for less surface area, and the dressing reaches the top parts of the salad. By the time the diner gets to the middle or end of the salad, there is little to no dressing left, making some add more fattening dressing. Spreading the salad out in a wider container or on a wider dish allows for the dressing to spread more and cover more salad.

Another option is to ask for a side of salsa! Depending on the salad combination, salsa can be a tasty and low/no fat dressing. Salsa is usually not considered because it is not listed in salad dressing choices. Most restaurants should have it; if they serve nachos, fajitas, burritos, and various appetizers, they will have salsa. Use that first and pour it on top of your salad. When there is barely any salsa left, about halfway through your salad, use the fattening dressing, but again, no more than two tablespoons. It is a great way to get a variety, two dressings in one meal. The salad will be coated more and you will enjoy more taste.

Be aware of the ingredients in the salad. If the salad has fattening ingredients mentioned such as fried chicken fingers and bacon, avoid it. Do not be afraid to make changes/requests. If the only "bad" ingredient is the fried chicken fingers, ask for grilled chicken instead. If beans are part of the salad, check to see if the beans are in oil or water. Simply ask! That can make a huge difference, as oil is of course very fattening. For instance, chick peas that I ordered for my salad were oily. I certainly learned my lesson that day. Do not be afraid to question; not everything can be assumed to be in its "healthy state."

Of course a safer option is to make your own salad at home. You know exactly what is going into it and do not have to question its content. But if making salad at home is not an option, dine out, but dine out smart using the tips and tricks I gave you!

CHAPTER 43

How to Keep the Deli Food DELIcious!

Perhaps some of you prefer to eat at a bagel shop or a café/deli. Most of these establishments serve generous helpings, especially when it comes to sandwiches. When I frequent these places for lunch, I have a system for each item:

Bagel and Cream Cheese

The cream cheese is obviously fattening. It also does not help when the layer of it on a bagel is about two inches high! This of course is overkill and there is more than needed for that cream cheese taste. Ask for the cream cheese on the side and lightly spread it on the bagel. Do not spread a thick layer. Spreading it thin will still accomplish that great taste. I like to spread the cream cheese on two bagel halves and then eat each half, one at a time. I will not bite into a whole bagel. The eating and tasting will last longer, keeping me more satisfied.

My son and I like to visit a favorite bagel shop. We have lunch together at this place quite a few times, especially during the summer. This one shop in particular gives so much cream cheese for bagel sandwiches, that we order one bagel with cream cheese, and one with nothing on it. I then delve into his cream cheese, lightly spreading some on my bagel. There was truly enough cream cheese on one sandwich that could really be applied to three bagels.

Sliced Meat and Cheese Sandwich

Before I give my tips on this, there is an important rule to follow. Avoid slathering on fattening spreads on the bread such as mayonnaise or butter. Try the sandwich without these first. Most of these meat and cheese sandwiches are served as a mega portion. Again, in a mega portion size world, cold cuts and such are piled high. The old me would eat everything that was on my plate. No portion of food was ever removed. At times things were added to the sandwich such as mayonnaise or a dressing of some sort. Never did I think to reduce my portion.

I make sure I have two pieces of meat and two pieces of cheese per sandwich. I take the remainder of the meat and cheese and ask for foil or plastic wrap so I could pack it and take it home to enjoy another day. Believe me, you will not miss it and you will still get the same taste.

Chicken Salad/Tuna Salad/Egg Salad Sandwiches

The fillings of these are obviously fattening. Most are loaded with mayonnaise. If it looks like there is more mayonnaise than tuna, for example, refrain from ordering it. If it is decent looking, either ask for the chicken, tuna, or egg salad on the side, or scrape it off of the sandwich and onto the plate. Take a spoon and take one scoop out from the mound of "salad" and put it on the bread. Feel free to take the leftovers home. Since these types of "salads" have mayonnaise, do not request a slathering of mayonnaise on the bread. Believe me, you have enough contained in the salad.

Requesting lettuce, tomato, onion, pickle, and pepper is perfectly fine.

Keep in mind that most restaurants pile on more food than one needs. Reducing what is in front of you will still allow you to enjoy your meal just as much as having all that piled up food. On the bright side, you will have extras to take home for another meal or snack. Be sure to bring a small insulated lunch bag with ice packs to bring the extras home. Those extras that you do bring home show your ability to have control over your portions!

CHAPTER 44

Avoid the Movie Crunch

It is fun to see a movie on the big screen. It is a way to escape the everyday "have to's" of our lives. Going to the movies is a great release, a fabulous diversion, but the food most of us choose to eat at the theater is not so great. The concession stand is extremely tough to resist. Once you walk into the movie theater lobby, the smell of freshly popped popcorn disseminates through the air. This aroma makes you want to buy something and munch away.

Sadly, a lot of movie theater food choices are not the best for our bodies. The popcorn is popped in oil, which makes it very fattening from the get go. Adding "butter," even just a little, makes it even worse. I put "butter" in quotes because oftentimes this "butter" is a chemical creation of anything but butter. Other choices aside from popcorn include candy, churros, nachos with cheese, hotdogs, pizza, and ice cream. I have never seen a movie theater offer fresh fruit or baked potato chips. Basically, the only things that are remotely healthy for selections are bottled water and 100% natural juices. Perhaps theaters do offer better choices, but there are none to be seen in my area.

The next time you go to the movies, think about whether or not you really need that food. Some of us do the "dinner and a movie" themed date night. After eating at a restaurant, is it highly necessary to have more food? Are you really that hungry? I personally think most people do not eat movie theater food because they are starving. It is a trained way to be, to munch something while at a theater. Additionally, the smells of the concession stand trick us into thinking that we are hungry.

We program ourselves to eat movie theater food, whether we are hungry or not. This scenario I see time and time again on cruise vacations, as described in the *Don't Get Your Money's Worth* chapter. After indulging on a multi course meal, most of us trek to the theater to see the evening's show. Almost all cruises have a performance soon after a specific dining time. I always see a great many people at the concession stand. Some I recognize from our dinner seating. They were able to have a multicourse meal, yet there they are, purchasing bags of popcorn, peanuts, and candy. They just had dinner! Serving sizes are generous and if wanted, a person can order as many entrees as he or she wishes. There are plenty of soups, salads, appetizers, huge entrees, and desserts. There is plenty of food to be had, yet there they were, making grand snack purchases. These people then try to perform a balancing act by gathering all the snacks and walking to their seats. This made me see that we snack not out of need, but because of routine. We are used to snacking during a movie or show, so we go through the motions and stuff our faces!

Most of the time I would go see a movie after a nice dinner. I would be full of course, but would purchase a large popcorn with lots of butter. Most of the time the popcorn was gone before the movie even started. Movie previews were longer and I ate fast! Sometimes I would have a box of candy or two. A large soda often accompanied my food. I used to be overly stuffed and did not feel so well. In retrospect, did I really need all of that or even any of that?

Timing is important in life, so I would suggest seeing a movie after a meal. You will be less likely to eat a lot. If you are famished, you will eat more. If you just finished a meal, you are less likely to eat as much.

I would also suggest refraining from eating during a movie. Most of the time we are eating out of habit. We are also paying attention to what is on the screen, whether it be the movie previews or the movie itself. We are not aware of what we are eating, and we feel unsatisfied. If you absolutely have to have something to snack on, I would recommend a kid's size popcorn without the "butter." Do not get a small size and assume you will share nicely with whoever you are with. Some people eat faster than others. I used to be one of those people, and would eat quickly. In reality, I would eat ¾ of the popcorn while my date ate a mere ¼ of the popcorn. Ordering a small size, especially a child's size popcorn, would be ideal. As a beverage, I would go for bottled water. Soda has lots of chemicals, and lots of calories. Even if it is a diet soda, it still has lots of chemicals. Avoid it at all costs!

If need be, you could gross yourself out by looking at the unhealthy food. See the chapter on grossing yourself out on the "bad" food. The hot dogs rotating under the neon lights look very unappetizing. Some food, especially those under the hot lamps, seem like they have been there all day. Who wants to eat that old food? The pizza looks like cardboard and is dried out under those bright lights.

Now that I told you how to handle the more traditional movie theaters, let me tell you how to handle the more "modern" movie theaters, which is a lot easier. At the time of this writing, dinner in the movie theater is becoming more prominent. It is like a restaurant in a movie theater, where servers bring food to your seat, and you get to enjoy a meal while watching a flick. This is more of restaurant food, so see the previous chapter on restaurant eating. The "rules" do apply. It is a nice treat and a fun experience, but I would not make it a habit to dine in a movie theater. Concentrating on the movie screen and not what is eaten can make one feel deprived. People do not realize how much food they consume during the movie and do feel cheated when the food is gone. They feel deprived and actually believe that they did not eat much at all. This leads to wanting more and overeating results.

You can really enjoy the movie without eating all that food. Most likely you are not hungry anyway. Curb the food and you will be even closer to getting to the new you! Cutting back a little can lead to huge changes in the end!

More cool stuff

CHAPTER 45

Losing Weight and Having Clothes-zure (Closure)

One thing you need to do is get rid of the big clothes. This is a major step because most of us do not want to do this. Perhaps we will gain the weight back as usual and need to have these back up clothes. Perhaps we can get "big bucks" by selling some of these gems. Another excuse is that some clothes have too much sentimental value.

The latter excuse was my biggest problem. One of the major gifts my mom would buy me was clothes. For every holiday, every occasion, or even a "just because I love you" reason, Mom would gift me clothes. We were so close; she was my mom, but also a sister and friend. She passed away in 2001 from a hellish battle with cancer. Just the idea of getting rid of the clothes she bought me would make me sick inside.

Ten years after her passing, I found myself with a major problem. My closet was getting out of control. Clothes were packed in to a point where I could not find things easily. The closet was a sloppy mess as well, with piles of clothes starting to amass on the floor. There were various shirt sizes: medium, large, extra large, 2X, 3X. There were also various pants sizes: 6, 8, 10, 12, 14, 16, 18, 20, 22, 24,

26. Many were either out of style or were not to my liking anymore. For instance, many of the pants were elastic, and I now detest wearing elastic pants. Some styles were to conceal bulges, so I no longer wished to wear those types of clothes. Besides, most of those were too big on me anyway. At this point, a charitable organization sent me a post card about a clothing drive. I finally made my move and called. Pickup was to be in fourteen days. This gave me plenty of time during the Christmas holiday season. Putting certain items in bags broke my heart. There was a queasiness feeling in my gut, but this was something I had to do. My clothes were getting out of hand. Also, for me, this was another way to stick to my healthy eating. I no longer had the security or back up of larger sizes. I am not wealthy, so buying a whole new wardrobe to accommodate a larger me was not an option. Saving the clothes to sell on the internet or elsewhere is not realistic. I wouldn't have time to itemize every article of clothing. Even if this was the only job I had, there would honestly not be enough hours in the day. People would not buy most of these clothes anyway. Giving away the large wardrobe did not only help my organization, but it gave me an extra reason to stay on track. Gaining weight was no longer an option. Eleven bags later, clothes were ready for the organization to give to the needy. So collectively, giving the clothes away helped organize my life, give me an extra excuse to stay on a healthy eating track, and give wonderful clothes to needy people.

I must admit, there were a few items of clothing I could not part with, but I do stress that there were a few items. Keeping a few articles helped me stay close to my mom in some way. Additionally, I took comfort in knowing that I have some of Mom's possessions that also help me keep close to her. For instance, I always wear one piece of her jewelry everyday so I can be close to her all day. Therefore, I am always wearing something from her. So the clothes are not the only thing I need - there are other items that I can treasure. Of course material things are not the most essential; I realize that the wonderful memories of the times we had together are most important. Additionally, I kept a few large tops that were shrunk a bit over time and still fit fine. I kept a few size 2X and 3X tee shirts to use as nightgowns/nightshirts. So these items remained for some use or sentimental value while everything else sadly had to go.

Regardless of your emotional ties or fears of gaining, give away most of these large size clothes. It is a good feeling to get rid of the larger sizes, and it is wonderful to help those who are less fortunate. If you have the time to sell nicer clothes, do try selling them on the internet or through a consignment shop. Most of us do not have the time to do these things, but if by chance you do, go for it. If time to gather clothes is an issue, keep a bag in your closet and pledge each day to put one article of clothing you do not need into it. Over time, it will add up and you will have enough to give away. Keep in mind that you will not have a backup set of clothes available if you should fall off the healthy eating wagon. This factor alone should keep you on track. It sure is keeping me on track. If I "grow out" of my clothes, there is nothing to fit into!

CHAPTER 46

Why It Sucks To Be Thin(ner)

I thought it would only be fair to discuss the negative aspects of being thinner. Many good things have some drawbacks. Here is my list:

You will have to purchase smaller sizes. Gee, what a terrible thing! You have to buy clothes that are a smaller size! Though it is an added expense, I would be more than happy to buy a small size instead of a 3X or size 26 jeans. It is obviously better to wear a smaller size than a larger size. And as you know, this will lead to cleaning out the closet.

Pessimists will be jealous. Some people cannot be happy for others. They must always put a negative spin on things, or say vitriolic comments out of jealousy. Remember, you have the upper hand. You have something that they want, and they will not get it, especially with that negative attitude and lack of positive spirit.

Well as you can see, my list of why it sucks to be thin is much shorter than the *Why it Sucks to be Fat* list. The latter was pages and pages longer. Can you see which is better? Are you ready to make the change? Did you take notes to help you with a game plan? I sincerely hope so. So go out there and be a better person, physically and mentally!

CHAPTER 47
Photos of Shame and Victory

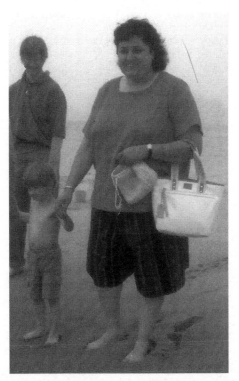

My son, husband, and I at the beach in June 2007. This was just a couple of weeks before my car accident, which even added more weight to this already huge frame. A group of family members asked me to join them for a walk along the beach. I remember trying to walk through the sand, huffing and puffing. I was lagging behind, unable to keep up.

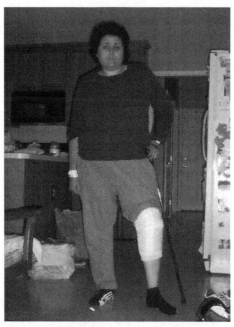

This picture was just taken after one of my knee surgeries, a result of a car accident that was not my fault. I was obese, in pain, and completely miserable. This was one of the lowest points in my life. I felt like a complete failure. I did lose a few pounds between the time I had the car accident and this knee surgery, but it is clear that I had a long way to go.

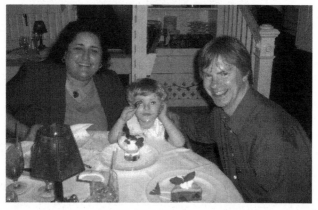

Having a nice dinner with my family. I was at 272 pounds in this picture, probably more after the multi-course meal I ate. The end result of a great meal was always the same. I was stuffed, fatigued, and disappointed in myself.

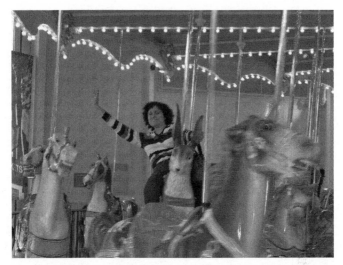

Enjoying one of the fruits of my labor. Look! I can ride the merry-go- round without having to worry about a weight restriction!

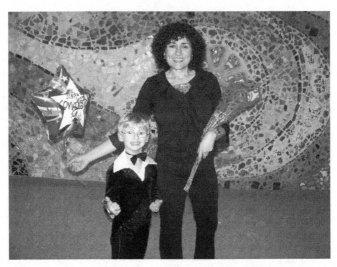

This picture was taken after our dance recital. I danced tap and my son was in tap and jazz numbers for his age group. It was special that we could both be in the same dance recital. I felt so youthful! It was a huge celebration. We went to an ice cream parlor afterwards where I had three scoops of chocolate ice cream with hot fudge, wet walnuts, caramel, marshmallow topping, chocolate chips, M&Ms...just kidding! We actually went straight home because it was late. We did go out to lunch the next day to celebrate and I had a <u>sensible</u> meal!

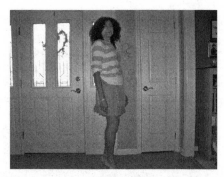

The outfit I "earned" and got to wear on *The Rachael Ray Show*. It was a modeling opportunity of a lifetime! I loved the outfit but was not too thrilled with this disheveled look! I just got off the train, picked my son up from after care in school, and drove an hour in traffic. It was hot that day and I was overheated in that sweater after getting out of the studio! Regardless, it was a fun day that I will remember for the rest of my life!

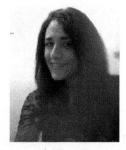

Feeling good about myself, I decided to step up my workout clothes and regular wardrobe. I even changed my hairstyle completely!

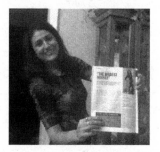

My first major article! *Oxygen Magazine* titled me "The Biggest Winner" in May 2014. The article well captured my struggles with weight and bullying. I did not realize at the time that this was the start of more articles to come!

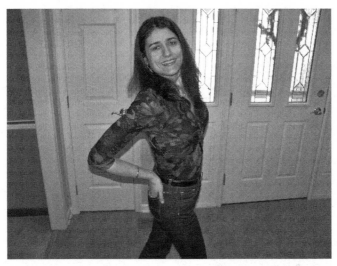

One of my favorite pictures and one of my favorite pairs of Lucky Brand jeans!

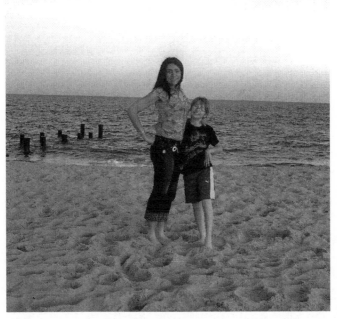

My son Joseph and me at the beach. I am equipped with a pedometer to track my steps and make sure I do my set minimum each day. Another fruit of my labor is that I can now proudly walk on the beach, and with ease. It is no longer an arduous activity. My ability is not stifled anymore and I feel more free!

CHAPTER 48

A Huge Fruit of My Labor

As most struggling authors know, it is an absolute must to have some sort of fame, some sort of platform in order for a literary agent to be interested. Therefore, my plan was to hit the talk show circuit, and tell my story of struggle and success. I emailed all the major talk shows and morning shows. There was no response, no interest. Such "silence" made me want to quit then and there. It was a downer and was very frustrating. Why didn't anyone want to see me? Wasn't my story interesting enough?

Just when I was ready to surrender my dream, I saw a big sign at my local Barnes and Noble, announcing a major book signing. Rachael Ray was going to autograph copies of her new burger book. It was the perfect opportunity to try to get on her show. Instead of my requests getting lost in the sea of emails, I could get direct contact with the show's host.

It was a tedious process on that special day. First, there was a line at the bookstore to get wrist bands. This granted a place in line. It was best to show up before the 4 o'clock distribution. What if they ran out of wrist bands? For me, there was no taking chances. I had come this far, so I got on line early and received a wrist band.

The next line was to wait for the actual book signing. The original plan was to meet my husband nearby so he could take my eight year old son, who was with me all day, to dancing school. As I saw the line grow, I begged my husband to meet us on the line. Fortunately my gracious and accommodating husband agreed. In the meantime, my son was kept busy with the iPod and I was paging through the newly purchased book I bought for Rachael to sign. What tremendous recipes in *The Book of Burger*. I was reading and planning.

While waiting in line, I heard a voice addressing people behind me. The woman introduced herself as a reporter for the *Trenton Times*. She wanted to find out tidbits about the fans so she could write a story about the book signing. *What brings you here? How long have you been a fan of Rachael Ray's?* I heard responses. I am not one to promote myself, so it was my hope that the reporter would approach me. But what if she didn't come to me? It would be a lost opportunity. With all the courage I could muster, I tapped the reporter's arm. She looked at me and I locked into her stare.

"I have a good story for you," I promised with confidence. The reporter saw the seriousness in my face and knew I meant business. She came closer with pen and pad in hand.

I told her about my weight loss and her eyes widened. To validate my claim, I pulled out the "before" pictures of an obese, wide me. Her eyes widened further. The reporter asked me several questions. Then people standing in line around us asked questions. One asked me about buying a new wardrobe after such a weight loss.

"It is an absolute thrill to find my size," I said with glee. When I was a size 3X and a size 26 jeans, I couldn't find my size in most stores and had to order from a catalogue. Now I'm a size medium and size 6 jeans (back then - now I am a size small and size 4 jeans). I also love wearing clothes I would never wear when I was obese, like tank tops and belts.

There was much congratulations, as well as kind words. For a brief moment, I felt famous. Throughout my life, I was put down.

I was always the wrong color, wrong religion, wrong size. Now I was seen as a person with value, a person who accomplished something. I was a "non-loser." My son looked on with such pride. How fortunate he was to see the "winning me" and people who actually gave me honor and respect. At that point, the reporter announced, "Remember the name, Lori Sweeney. She's going to be famous someday!"

The rest of the time on line was filled with silence and chatter. Sometimes I stood quiet, and sometimes I chatted with my son or the woman next to me. Nervousness rose as the time got closer to meet Rachael Ray.

"I heard she's not as nice as she is on TV," one voice said. This made the nervousness become panic.

"Oh, I heard she is very nice to work for," another voice said. A wave of calm came over me, and I breathed a sigh of relief.

My husband arrived to take my son to dancing school. By then there were two lines with about 400 people waiting. How fortunate I was to make a good decision. Had I left the line to drop off my son, my chances of meeting Rachael Ray could have been dashed. My son and husband wished me luck as I was left to face this opportunity alone.

Finally, my time came. The line moved gradually and Rachael Ray came into my view. Incredible! Her sweet face and her kind demeanor to those ahead of me relieved my anxiety. There was no more fear in asking. When it was my turn, I told Rachael while she was signing my book that I was in her studio audience a year ago. Rachael responded with information that the studio was moving to a new location.

"I have something cool to show you," I said. With that, I pulled out the "before" pictures and spread them out in front of her. Rachael looked down at them and then looked at me; her eyes widened. Quite honestly, I cannot remember the exact wording she used, but it was something to the effect of, "Wow, you look amazing!"

"And I did it all myself - that's why it worked."

I handed her a small, laminated page that had "before" and "after" shots of me. I included contact information and interesting bullet points. I told her I would love to be on her show. Rachael in turn wrote a name on the paper and handed it to her assistant.

"This person is in charge of our weight loss stories," she said. "We are now on hiatus, but if we're interested, we'll contact you in the fall. In the meantime, come see our new studio."

"I shall! Thank you Rachael," I said. I left with happiness in my heart, accomplishing more than what I thought possible.

The next morning, I eagerly searched the internet for the story. The article was easily found. I was reading and reading, while simultaneously reliving the wonderful memories in my head. I was not 100% sure I would find my name in the article. It looked like the reporter had conducted many interviews and had a multitude to choose from. I then came across a one sentence mention that I was an excited individual who wanted to show Rachael Ray photos of my weight loss and to be a guest on her show.

"I made the internet! I made the internet!" I screamed. My husband and son came from different directions to see for themselves. My husband appeared to be in shock. My son jumped up and down, and I joined him. I even did a little dance of my own. That one sentence in the paper made me more than elated. Such happiness drove me to run out with my son to purchase the actual newspaper. The article was in that day's edition and I found my name in print. We bought five out of the six copies, leaving a "courtesy copy" behind. I was that thrilled about a one sentence mention. Little did I know this was the beginning of many articles. Some would not just mention me in one sentence but would actually feature my story!

I showed my clients. Some were thrilled for me while others were stoic. A few mentioned that they hoped I would not get famous and quit tutoring. My husband later told me I should take that concern as a compliment. I tried but found myself considering the threads of selfishness woven through the intricate designs of life.

One friend emailed the link in case I did not know. Another person, a pseudo friend, informed me of the article as well. She always vows to get together but never follows through. A few weeks prior to the article, I reached out to her and she didn't even respond to my email. Yet, there she was-demanding tickets to see the show when I get to be a guest! This "user attitude" disgusts me for many reasons. First of all, it is a ridiculous request of someone who is not close to me. Secondly, I don't even know if I will be on the show. Thirdly, I am not in charge of tickets. Most importantly, if I got on the show, I would have to concern myself with things other than ensuring she gets a seat. In my response to her I explained that I'll find out in the fall if there is interest to feature me. I also advised her to contact the show via website to request seeing Lori Sweeney, who lost over 100 pounds as mentioned in the *Times* article. I never heard back from her. I also asked clients I considered to be close with to email *The Rachael Ray Show* and ask to feature me. Most declined, expressing their concerns about me leaving the tutoring business. Some flat out told me that they did not want me to be famous! A true friend of mine, Deepika, wrote to the show, saying I was an inspiration for her quest to lose weight. This meant the world to me; I was proud to be an inspiration to her. Additionally, I was grateful she made the effort to contact the show while others flat out refused.

The show contacted my friend; since she mentioned her weight loss struggles, the show wanted her for a weight loss segment. Though Deepika tried to plug me in the midst of the conversation, there was no interest in my story. A producer pressed forward and asked for photos, but decided she was not in the overweight range they were looking for. The producer still liked her and wanted Deepika's participation in some kind of segment. Finally, she was going to be in a jeans segment and asked me to accompany her for the fitting the day before the show. Deepika thought it would be a great opportunity to schmooze the staff members and drum up interest. (Don't we all wish to have more good friends like her?) I did do the schmoozing but found my category was not going to be covered in the near future. Therefore, my self-promotion was pointless. That is show business, I guess! After the fitting, Deepika asked a producer if I could join her in the studio for filming day so she wouldn't have to travel in alone.

"Sure," the producer said. She then looked right at me. "To give you a heads up, you will be in a back room and won't be in the audience because we are all booked. A lot of people who accompany our guests think they will be in the audience, so I didn't want it to be a surprise." She was kind to tell the truth, but I was still willing to attend. I knew I would be in an isolated room, having little contact with staff. I pitched my case and there was nothing further to do. I was there for my friend, solely for moral support and for company. I wanted to make sure that she would not have to travel alone. It was not about me anymore. As open as I am, I had to let Deepika know the truth.

"Just so you know, I want to join you to support you," I said. "I am not out to promote myself further. I did my "schpiel," got myself out there, and now it is up to them. I am here for you. If I'm going to sit in a back room, I'll bring work and call back some clients." Deepika told me she understood and she knew I was there solely for her.

So there I was, up again at four in the morning as I was the day before the taping. Robert was going to take Joseph to school. Though I was not going to be in the studio audience and was going to be hidden backstage, I still dressed nicely out of respect. I wanted to look decent, even though I was to sit in a dark corner of the backstage. I met Deepika at her house and we rode together to the train station.

My job was to psyche up Deepika. I called her a soon-to-be superstar. We were both very excited. Her phone rang while we were on the train to New York. It was a producer from the show. I thought the call was about last minute directions or questions to help shape the show, so I tuned out of the conversation. My head was filled with who to call and what work to do in my spare time. Deepika soon handed me the phone.

"They want to talk to you," Deepika said with a grin. I felt the electrical shock of adrenalin rush through me.

An effervescent producer, Monica, told me that she is working on a piece called "Lucky 13," 31 looks utilizing 13 articles of clothing. A total of 31 women were modeling. One called out sick and she was looking for a replacement.

"Are you around a size 6 or 8?" Monica asked.

"I'm a size 6," I cheerfully responded. I would be a perfect fit - and I was. This was amazing to me. If I hadn't lost the weight, I would not be in the segment. If I didn't lose the weight, Deepika would not be in her segment. It was her writing on my behalf that helped her get on the show. And it was my selfless support that brought me to the right place at the right time. After hearing the arrangements, I returned the phone to Deepika with my mouth agape.

"I'm going to be a model!" I cried.

After filling her in, we both got busy on our cell phones. I called Robert, who is a very mellow, unexcitable man. I knew I made it to the big time when he cracked his coolness. He spoke excitedly and his voice got high. Deepika called her husband and texted many of our friends. Indeed it was amazing karma. We both tried to help each other and both got on the show. Though it wasn't the segment I'd envisioned when telling my weight loss success story, I was grateful to be on the show. It sounded like fun and it was a guaranteed appearance. I decided to take the gift I was given and make something out of it. Perhaps using this appearance would get literary agents interested.

We arrived at the studio to discover a line of people waiting to be part of the studio audience. A staff member was waiting for us, and, like VIP's, we were escorted in right into the building; that alone made me feel special. Because of the different segments, Deepika and I had to be split up. Unfortunately I wouldn't be there to give her support. We would spend the whole day not knowing about how the other was faring.

I was escorted into a room with 30 women. Many were confused to see the new person. After all, they had come the day before to try on outfits I told my story to all who asked; many could not believe my good fortune. Some confessed that they thought the producer called in a professional model to fill in. Imagine! I looked like a model to them! If they only knew where I came from!

Though there were many people, the place was very organized. Clothes were hanging neatly, with multiple styles in multiple sizes. My size, even in shoes, was waiting for me. Because I was "new," I had to try on a couple of outfits. I liked the way I looked in each one. This made my weight loss even "sweeter." The day was packed with lots to do; we did a dress rehearsal so we could understand positioning. We had hair and makeup done. Employees came to inspect us and accessorize. Some of us received pocketbooks, clutches, scarves, or earrings. It was a fun experience. I ended up wearing a light colored sweater, a light pink skirt, and beige high heels.

Throughout it all, staff members had the patience of saints. There were so many needs among 31 women. Two had to have their tattoos covered by makeup. A few needed their clothes steamed to get the wrinkles out. Others needed their skirts pinned. I needed a new bra! I wore a red bra, not knowing my fate for that day. The light colored sweater would allow the red bra to show through easily. I alerted a segment coordinator, gave my size, and in a snap, got just the right bra. It was magical; just request something and poof, it was there!

We were finally led backstage. I heard the warm up guy psyching up the audience with his jokes. Rachael Ray came out to personally greet the studio audience. They were ready to film. We heard the intro music and later on heard our cue. Soon, I found myself strutting out like a model. So there I was, standing in front of a cheering audience. I was able to show off the fruits of my labor to the television world. It was a rare opportunity; this idea raced through my head as the audience and cameras faced me. Pride and comfort came upon me. I was not the loser who people saw from years ago. I did not hang my head down in shame that day as I did for most of my young life. I was a winner, a star in my own right. Those people who didn't believe in me, those who couldn't treat me decently could eat their hearts out! I am sure they would never think I could be anything great. I was Isla, I was Fatness. But there I was, posing on a sound stage in front of the cameras. I was able to radiate with joy after years of being stomped on, not being allowed to shine.

I tried to be the best model I could be, which later concerned me. Many of the ladies turned to Rachael Ray as she spoke with the fashion coordinator during the segment. I looked straight ahead, just like the models on the shopping networks. I would have moved around, but I was sandwiched between two ladies. I looked straight ahead and smiled, trying to be the most professional "model." I posed so sexy that Rachael called me "saucy." I so wanted to react to the amazing comment, but I kept on posing. Staying focused and not interacting with the show host made me question how I looked later on. It was not fear that made me frozen, it was the idea to pose like a model that had me fixated where I was, beaming with pride!

After our segment, we got to sit in the audience and watch the rest of the filming. It was a fabulous experience. I still could not believe I was on a major television show and that I got to stick around to watch the rest of the fun! At the same time, I wondered where Deepika was. She surely was finished with her segment.

After the taping we all gathered up our things. I thanked the staff who worked closely with us. They worked their hearts out for sheer perfection. A staff member approached me and connected me with Deepika. She was in the green room, watching our segment. She enjoyed it, as well as her experience. We spent the train ride recalling about our experiences. It was an amazing day for both of us.

I went to Joseph's school right away to pick him up from the after school program. I told him the surprising news. Joseph jumped up and down as if we'd won the lottery. He jumped and hugged, jumped some more, hugged some more. I was excited as well. With all that excitement, we decided to go to a supermarket to pick up prepared foods for dinner. After an exciting day, I was too exhausted to cook. With every supermarket staff member we encountered, Joseph would say, "Tell them the good news!" He was so thrilled for me and it was like a dream!

We had a nice meal. Robert came home and I filled him in on the details. I made a few more calls to share the good news with friends. When it was time to get to bed, I cannot even remember my head hitting the pillow; I think I fell asleep in the midst of plopping down on the bed.

When I woke up, I was still bubbling with excitement. I reflected on that special day and still could not believe what had happened to me. It was my hope that this would be a turning point in my journey and that I would be able to somehow get my tips, tricks, and message across. I wanted to inspire others to get healthier, creating their own success.

After spending weeks skimming *The Rachael Ray Show* website for upcoming shows, I spotted my airdate. As a bonus, a picture was posted on the site that had me standing in the back. I had five days to pull things together. The 60-plus literary agents who I emailed previously needed to be updated on my television appearance. Perhaps my news would make me more appealing to work with. Friends, clients, and relatives needed to be told.

Reactions were very surprising. Literary agents didn't care at all. Some people were excited for me, you might have thought they were going to be on television. Others showed little to no interest. Whether it was a friend or client, I always took interest in their lives. I was a good listener and rarely jumped in with information about my own life. Now I shared good news and few were interested. Regardless of reaction, I continued to spread the good news.

Everything came into place and soon it was time for my big premiere. Robert took the morning off so we could watch it together. My television was set to record the show for Joseph to see. As the show's airing time approached, the air itself became very thin. It was quite difficult for me to breathe. Once the show started, our eyes were glued to the set. Soon it was time for the models to come out - and there I was! I was shocked to see myself up there, tall and thin. Rachael called me "saucy." She liked the saucy one in the middle! It was a wonderful way to unexpectedly celebrate my major weight loss accomplishment.

When the segment was over, the fun and surprises did not end. The remaining segments were interesting. About halfway into the show, there were camera shots of me in the audience. From that point on, I was shown a total of five additional times. It was a shock, as well as an honor. Joseph loved it when I showed him the video.

He kept kissing me because he was so proud of his mom. With that much love and respect, it made losing 125 pounds even sweeter.

The end of that episode of *The Rachael Ray Show* summed it up. Before the show ended, there was a shot of me in the studio audience clapping, and mouthing "wow." That scene says it all. It was a wow, a <u>big</u> wow. A loser in my childhood, I rose to become a fit, trim, and confident human being who wishes to help others. The naysayers in my life tried to put me down, but I spent most of my life trying to bring people up! My weight loss goal was to initially make my life easier; it was such a struggle to carry around such weight and find clothes that would fit me. My achievements have motivated others. And that is not all; I got to model for a major television show. Looking at where I came from, what I have now morphed into, and where I ended up, is a major, wondrous "Wow!"

Deepika's segment aired days later and turned out fabulous! We supported each other and were proud of our appearances. It was amazing what the powers of friendship and perseverance can do!

CHAPTER 49

My Life Now/Afterward

It has been a long journey, but a fruitful one. Losing weight was one of the best, most successful things I have done. It has reduced my problems and given me so many bonuses in my life. I no longer get up from a meal overstuffed and fatigued. I can do whatever physical labor I need to do without huffing and puffing. I can keep up with my son, one of my biggest supporters during this weight loss journey. Very importantly, I can keep up with my family as a whole, participating in activities instead of sending them on their way to have fun without me. Clothes in my size are in abundance, and I have a true choice of what to wear. My size small shirt and my size 4 jeans can easily be found in stores. There is no more digging to the bottom of the clothes pile to find a 3X in any store (if the store even carried the 3X size)! I can explore fashion and wear things I did not feel comfortable wearing before such as belts, bikini underwear, tank tops, short shorts, dresses, and bathing suits. I no longer have to pay a premium for a larger size. I can look at myself in the mirror without the disgust that I had another failing day of trying to lose weight. I can look down and see my legs, not my stomach. When I was over 250 pounds, my stomach blocked my upper thigh. In addition to all the mentioned benefits, one of the most important advantages is that I get to spread my advice and reach more people through this book. I enjoy many areas of teaching; educating in this way is indeed very fruitful and satisfying. It is tutoring on a wider scale!

I can easily look at the naysayers in my life and not look down. I can stare them right in the eyes and not be ashamed. These people mocked me and made sure to offer degrading comments about my weight. I am in better shape that these cretins and it feels good. Please do not feel I measure myself against everyone I meet. I only feel this way towards those who ridiculed me and looked down on me. If I see an overweight or obese person in public, I do make assumptions. Everyone has a reason why his or her body shape is the way it is. Laziness is not always the cause. When I do see an overweight or obese person, I do not judge. Sometimes I say to myself, "Gee, I think I can really help them. I can at least make them lose some of the weight, and losing some would be an overall improvement." I have been in their shoes. I know how it is. I do not even like it when people make fun of my "old me" pictures. That person used to be me and there are many who look as I did at 272 pounds. There is compassion I feel for others, whether large or small. The only exception is the group of poisonous people who made tremendous efforts to be unkind when they could have easily just walked without uttering one cruel word.

Strangely enough, looking back to the past and remembering the insults gives me such strength. When belittled, I gradually rose to be the person I always wanted to become, both on a physical and spiritual level. I did not let people or my weight keep me down. Therefore, losing weight tastes sweeter than any dessert I can eat.

Aside from looking at naysayers, I can actually look at myself. In the old days, I merely glanced at myself in the mirror or a shop window, not being able to stand what I saw. My unhappiness resided with my double chins, overstuffed face, and stomach hanging down to my knees. This was not the way I wanted to be. Now I do not mind seeing myself in the mirror. My look is still new to me. My face lost a chin and its stuffing. It is a more chiseled, sculpted face. My stomach does not hang over my knees. My legs are much thinner. Because being thinner is still a novelty, I catch myself staring in mall windows to see my reflection. Looking at myself may seem a bit vain, but I assure you it is not. It is a version of me that is so different. After years of being overweight, I am now a normal weight. This is a different view. I never stayed a healthy weight long enough to appreciate the change. My "new me" is still new to me. I never looked like this before and am still surprised.

The new me is also new to many people who know me. People who have not seen me for a while do not recognize me. I sometimes I have to reintroduce myself to these people and they are shocked to see that it is me. One time I was thrilled that a certain someone did not see me. An old coworker from my corporate life was sitting at a table diagonal from ours. She was a backstabber who betrayed our friendship once I accepted a job at another company. She did not notice me, and I was free and clear of being recognized. This anonymity was an added bonus to losing a great deal of weight; my "enemy" did not even recognize me and I did not wish to be recognized.

Losing weight has given me so much freedom. Confidence has taken its place. Dancing is now a part of my life. When I had a little bit of spare time, I did an adult tap dance for two recitals. No one made fun of me at all. I was not the dancing joke but was regarded as one of the top dancers in the group. I also have the freedom to do a variety of exercises which gives me pride, especially when I master such. I gained the confidence to model on *The Rachael Ray Show* without fear. I have the freedom to ride theme park rides without having to look at the weight restrictions. I have the freedom to wear clothes I was too afraid to wear. It was a thrill to wear a cute, stylish tank top on the boardwalk. I felt beautiful when I wore a strapless dress to a fancy dinner. I can even wear high heels. The old me could not keep my balance in them. My tremendous weight prevented me from accomplishing that. Additionally, I was afraid to wear a thin heel in fear that my weight would cause it to snap. Now I can wear a variety of heels without worry. And I do not mind strolls on the beach because I can actually walk in the sand with ease. The bottom line is that there is more freedom to do more things, and to even wear more things with confidence. For all of this I am truly grateful.

A big achievement for me was climbing the Cape May Lighthouse. It has 199 steps, a definite obstacle for a 200+ pound person. Years ago, I had to take breaks on the landings, trying to catch my breath along the way. It took a long time to reach the top and I barely made it up all those steps. The new me, the more fit me, was able to climb to the top without rest. To reach the top was exhilarating, a major accomplishment. Perhaps to some it is no big deal. Others have climbed major mountains. However, this was the mountain that the obese me could not climb with ease.

The looks of surprise when old clients or friends see me indicates the magnitude of my accomplishment. Some see me in a store and are afraid to approach me, fearing they are mistaken in assuming it is me. One admitted to saying aloud, "Is that Lori Sweeney?" so it would grab my attention if I was indeed the Lori Sweeney. Some said they were not sure it was me until they heard me speaking to a clerk. I have returned to some clients years later to tutor a younger child. How surprised they are to see me on their doorstep. Such looks of shock send a message to me that the differences are significant and that I really did something amazing here.

Losing weight has helped me set an example. I have been able to motivate through magazines, newspapers, and the internet. I made it on the front page of *The Star Ledger*, one of New Jersey's largest newspapers. I got a two page story. *The Hillsborough Beacon* did a great story on me as did Shapefit.com. *Oxygen Magazine* called me "The Biggest Winner." Without sounding conceited, which I am not, I am truly a winner. I figured it all out and took off the weight. I motivate people so they do not suffer as I did when I was trapped in an obese body. I build up people, and not tear them down, whether in this setting or as a tutor. People cheer me on and are motivated to improve themselves. Many have, and they make sure to inform me of their progress. How wonderful it is to see their transformations! I left corporate life for teaching and tutoring. It was my hope to educate and help others, and I am able to do so on a larger scale through this book.

No diet plan worked for me 100%. The stresses and lures of everyday life would break my dieting, causing me to "fall off the wagon." A string of eating holidays would make me quit. A string of stresses would make me eat and eat. Hosting dinners would make me forget about dieting. My responses to certain stimuli caused me to fail miserably at losing weight over the years. It took my plan, my ideas to teach me how to handle food better, to handle myself better. I wasn't "born" thin and many members of my family were not thin. I am an average person, so if I could do it, you can as well. If you took notes along the way and make plans to change, you can be just as successful.

Similar victories can be yours if you put in the effort. You will see the fruits of labor after weight loss. You will feel great about your accomplishments. The right people will give you accolades for your efforts. And filter out the unkind words from the wrong people! A major mistake I made was internalizing everything that was said, believing all unkind statements. The bottom line is that these people were not the experts in "loserology" and had their own issues. I am not the loser, the fatso, Isla, or other horrible names. And my name is not Fatness.

For everybody, losing weight can be a different experience. You will find your own rewards and unique positive experiences. So what are you waiting for? Find your new life! Go out and do it! Be honest with yourself, try, and persevere!

CHAPTER 50

Ravishing Recipes

There are other recipes found throughout the book, but as promised, here are some simple low fat or lower fat meals that I serve. If there is interest, I will publish low fat and low calorie recipes that I created myself. I utilized my old chemist skills and came up with recipes that are inspired by many cultures. I have so many recipes to share and these of course are just samplings. All recipes incorporate natural ingredients. For instance, I do not utilize sugar substitutes or other chemical concoctions. Feel free to make these for parties or simply enjoy the recipes for yourself!

All calories and fat values are approximate.

Hummus
(makes 10 servings – 90 calories and 5.2 g fat per serving)

- 1 can chick peas/garbanzo beans, drained
- 1 clove garlic
- 3 tbs lemon juice
- 2 tsp lemon zest
- 2 tbsp tahini/sesame paste
- 2 tsp 0% fat plain Greek yogurt
- ¼ tsp cumin
- ½ tsp salt
- parsley, cilantro, paprika - optional

Put all in a blender. Pulse until creamy. Can top with parsley and cilantro. Can lightly dust with paprika.

Feta Dumplings
(makes 12 servings – 90 calories and 2 g fat per serving)

Dough
- 1 ½ cups flour
- 1 tsp baking powder
- ½ cup 2% Greek yogurt
- 1 egg
- 2 egg whites
- 1 tbs sugar

Filling
- ½ cup feta cheese
- 2 tbs tahini
- 1 tsp cumin

Mix dough ingredients until uniform. Roll dough into balls. Flatten and push/indent in center of each with thumb. Mix filling ingredients together and spoon mixture in center of indents. Fold edges up, over top, pinching the top.

Bake at 350° for 20 minutes. Makes 12 servings/dumplings.

Chicken Parmesan
(makes 3 servings - 400 calories and 6 g fat per serving)

Ingredients

- egg whites - beaten. Start with 5, then beat more when needed. It depends on how much chicken you end up making.
- 1 lb raw chicken breast sliced
- 1 cup Italian seasoned bread crumbs
- ¼ cup parmesan cheese
- ½ cup of your favorite pasta sauce

Mix bread crumbs and parmesan cheese in a bowl and set aside. Dip chicken breasts in well beat egg whites. Then dip egg white coated chicken breasts in the bread crumb/parmesan cheese mixture, evenly coating both sides. Place coated chicken breasts on a prepped cookie sheet (layer of aluminum foil with a non stick spray applied). Bake at 375° for 15 minutes on each side. Top with two tablespoons of pasta sauce and bake for another five minutes.

Stuffed Shells
(for three shells, 350 calories, 9 g fat)

I usually have three stuffed shells. That would be my typical serving. Serve these buffet style and let people take as many as they wish.

Ingredients

- 1 box of jumbo shells pasta
- 1 lb part skim ricotta cheese
- ½ cup parmesan cheese or parmesan/romano cheese mixture - grated
- 1 package shredded mozzarella cheese.
- 1 jar of your favorite pasta sauce

Preheat oven to 375°

Put entire contents of ricotta cheese in a large bowl. Add grated cheese. Mix well and set aside.

Bring a large pot of water to a boil. Make sure pot is large enough to accommodate the shells to be cooked. Add shells and cook for 20 minutes. Test shells to determine sufficient cooking by sampling a small piece of a broken one (believe me, there will be broken ones by the time cooking is complete).

When cooking is complete, rinse the shells with cold water so they are easy to handle. Place on in a large spoon with open side up. This is the "platform" to do the stuffing. Stuff shell with one tablespoon of the ricotta/grated cheese mixture. Place each shell in a baking dish that was treated with cooking/nonstick spray. Put one tablespoon of pasta sauce over each shell. Place a half a tablespoon of shredded mozzarella over each shell. Bake for 20 minutes at 375°.

Simple Fruit Pie
(makes 8 servings - 125 calories, 1 g fat per serving)

- 1 circle of refrigerated pie crust dough
- 1 pie pan, about 8 inches in diameter
- 1 apple - washed and thinly sliced
- ½ cup strawberries - washed, green top off, thinly sliced
- ½ cup raspberries - washed, whole
- 1 can cooking spray
- 1 tbs sugar

Preheat oven to 375° . Spray pie pan with cooking spray to avoid food sticking to the pan. Center pie crust dough in pan, pressing dough into pan. Pie crust edges should be hanging over the pan. Add apples, placing them evenly on the pie crust. Add remaining fruit, distributing evenly. Fold up edges, overlapping fruit. The center of the pie should be open with just flaps of pie crust on the edges. Bake for one hour. Remove from oven and let sit 10 minutes. Serve and enjoy.

Cup of Joe Chocodoughnuts
(makes 15 doughnuts - 100 calories, 2.5 g of fat)

Dry Ingredients
- 2 cups flour
- 1 tbs baking powder
- 2 tsp cinnamon sugar
- ¼ tsp cloves

Liquid mixture
- ½ cup strong coffee, fresh and hot
- ½ cup chocolate chips

- ½ cup 2% Greek yogurt
- 1 egg
- 1 egg white
- 2 tsp vanilla extract
- ½ cup milk

Mix dry ingredients and set aside. Measure coffee and pour into chocolate chips. Stir until chips are melted. Add remaining liquid ingredients to this mixture. Add this complete liquid mixture to the dry mixture. Mix well. Pour into doughnut pans (makes 15 doughnuts) and bake at 350° for 20 minutes.

Whey Cool Cherry Smoothie
Makes two servings (130 calories and 1.5 grams of fat per serving)

Ingredients

- ½ cup 2% milk
- 1 cup frozen cherries
- 1 tbs dark chocolate cocoa powder
- 2 tbs vanilla whey protein
- ½ cup crushed ice (ice cubes if limited, but most refrigerators can dispense crushed ice)

Put all ingredients in a blender and blend for 20 to 30 seconds or blend on "smoothie" setting, if available. Pour in your favorite glass and enjoy!

Notes of Success

Use this guide to write down new ideas, the new tips/tricks you are going to try at each of the destinations. This really helps. **List what you will do differently for each destination and include a page number for reference!** I recommend photocopying it so you can utilize it again and again!

Core Luggage:

Home Luggage

Venturing out

Dining out

Traveling Game Plan

List your strategies for venturing out. Photocopy, fold, and bring this with you. Look at your notes accordingly so you know what to do when you venture out.

Work

Errands/Shopping

Vacation/Other

Restaurant/Party

Made in the USA
Lexington, KY
06 March 2016